PCOS DIET COOKBOOK

for Newly

Diagnosed

Flavorful polycystic Recipes

JAMMIE STONES

 DISCLAIMER 

TABLE OF CONTENT

Foreword

As a nutritionist specializing in women's health, I've had the privilege of witnessing countless transformations in the lives of those navigating the complex landscape of *Polycystic Ovary Syndrome (PCOS)*. I've seen the frustration, the uncertainty, and the fear that often accompany a diagnosis, but I've also seen incredible resilience, determination, and hope.

In this remarkable book, *"PCOS Diet Cookbook for the Newly Diagnose*d," **Jammie Stones** invites you into a world of flavor, nourishment, and empowerment. With meticulous attention to detail and a deep understanding of the challenges faced by those with PCOS, Jammie has crafted a comprehensive guide that goes beyond mere recipes—it's a roadmap to reclaiming your health and vitality.

Through her own journey and the stories of others, Jammie illustrates the transformative power of food, showing how simple, delicious meals can become potent tools for managing symptoms, regulating hormones, and improving fertility. Whether you're craving a comforting bowl of soup, a vibrant salad bursting with color, or a decadent dessert to satisfy your sweet tooth, you'll find inspiration on every page.

I wholeheartedly endorse this book as a valuable resource for anyone embarking on their PCOS journey. Let it be your companion, your confidant, and your culinary muse as you discover the joy of nourishing your body and nurturing your soul.

Warm regards,

Introduction

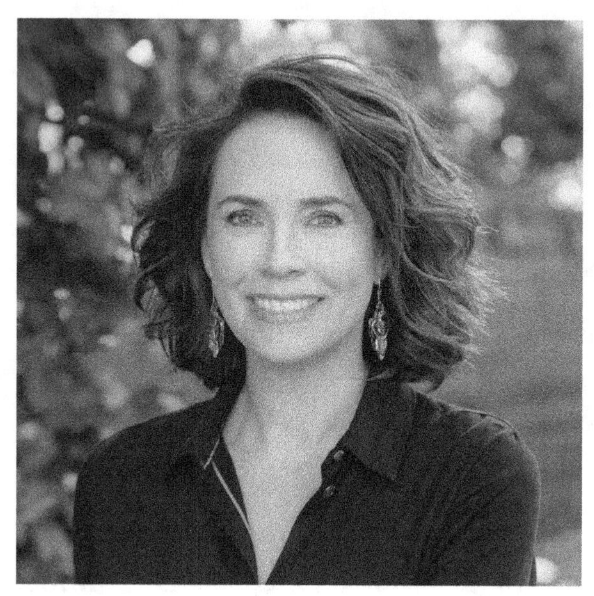

The Day My World Turned Upside Down (and How Food Became My Ally)

It all started with a simple question during my annual checkup. *"Have you noticed any irregular periods lately?"* My doctor's gaze held a concern that sent shivers down my spine. Uncharacteristically heavy periods had become a new normal, but I naively dismissed them as stress. Turns out, it was something more - PCOS.

The diagnosis felt like a punch in the gut. Images of weight gain, uncontrollable hair growth, and a struggle to conceive flooded my mind. I left the doctor's office feeling utterly lost. PCOS seemed like a monster under the bed, a thief stealing my control over my own body.

Determined to fight back, I dove headfirst into research. Countless articles and websites blurred together, but one message kept reappearing: **diet is a powerful tool in managing PCOS**. Skeptical but hopeful, I started exploring different meal plans. The world of PCOS diets felt overwhelming - low-carb, anti-inflammatory, vegan... where do I even begin?

That's when I realized there weren't many resources specifically designed for **newly diagnosed women like me**. We needed clear, easy-to-follow guidance that wasn't intimidating or restrictive. We needed recipes that were delicious and didn't feel like punishment. Most importantly, we needed to know we weren't alone.

This cookbook is my answer to that cry for help. It's the culmination of everything I've learned on my PCOS journey, from the initial shock to the small victories and everything in between. These recipes aren't just about managing symptoms; they're about reclaiming your health and celebrating your body.

They're the fuel that helped me transform my relationship with food. No longer the enemy, food became my biggest ally. It empowered me to take charge of my PCOS and live a life that wasn't dictated by the condition.

So, if you've just been diagnosed with PCOS, take a deep breath. You are not alone. *This book is your roadmap to a healthier, happier you.* Let's turn this diagnosis into an opportunity to discover the strength and resilience you never knew you had. Let's get cooking!

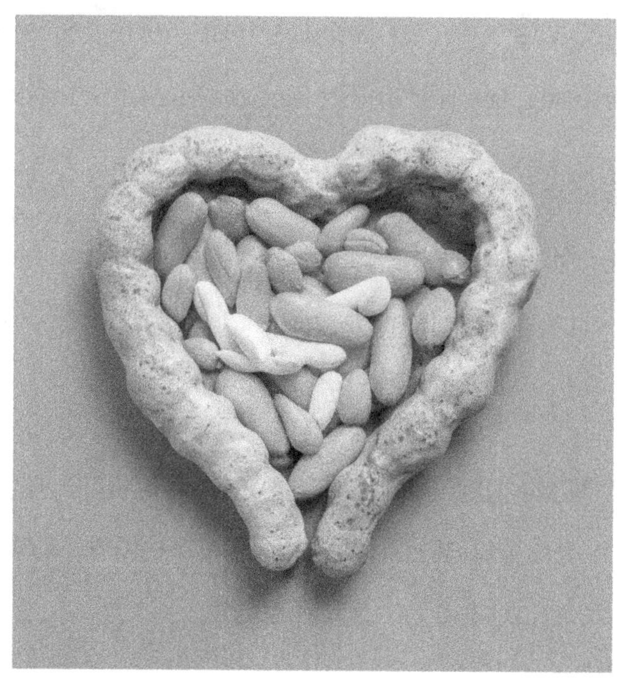

Chapter 1: Understanding PCOS

What is PCOS?

PCOS, which stands for Polycystic Ovary Syndrome, is a hormonal imbalance that affects women during their childbearing years. It's one of the most common endocrine disorders for women of reproductive age.

Here's a breakdown of what happens with PCOS:

- **Hormonal Imbalance:** Ovaries normally produce eggs and hormones like estrogen and progesterone to regulate your menstrual cycle. With PCOS, your ovaries produce higher-than-normal amounts of androgens, often referred to as "male" hormones, although women naturally have small amounts. This disrupts the balance and can lead to issues with ovulation.

- **Irregular Periods:** Since ovulation (egg release) may not happen regularly, periods become irregular or infrequent.

- **Cysts on Ovaries:** The name "polycystic" refers to the small cysts that may form on the ovaries. These contain immature eggs and don't always release them properly.

Some common symptoms of PCOS include:

- Irregular or missed periods
- Excess hair growth on the face and body (due to the androgen imbalance)
- Acne
- Weight gain or difficulty losing weight
- Difficulty getting pregnant

It's important to note that not everyone with PCOS will experience all of these symptoms, and the severity can vary.

If you're concerned you might have PCOS, talking to your doctor is the best course of action. They can help diagnose the condition and create a treatment plan tailored to your specific needs.

PCOS: Symptoms and Diagnosis

PCOS (Polycystic Ovary Syndrome) can present itself in a variety of ways, so it's important to be familiar with the common symptoms and how doctors typically diagnose the condition.

Symptoms:

- **Irregular Periods:** This is a hallmark symptom of PCOS. You may experience missed periods, infrequent periods (less than eight per year), or periods that last longer than a week.
- **Excess Androgen Levels:** Androgens are hormones typically associated with males, but females have them in small amounts too. PCOS can cause an imbalance, leading to symptoms like:
    - Increased facial and body hair growth (hirsutism)
    - Acne
    - Male-pattern baldness or thinning hair
- **Weight Gain or Difficulty Losing Weight:** PCOS can affect how your body processes insulin, a hormone that regulates blood sugar. This can lead to weight gain and make it harder to lose weight.
- **Skin Changes:** Oily skin and skin tags (small flaps of skin) on the neck or under the arms can be signs of PCOS.
- **Difficulty Getting Pregnant:** Irregular ovulation caused by PCOS can make it challenging to conceive.

It's important to remember that not everyone with PCOS will experience all of these symptoms, and the severity can vary greatly. Some women may only have mild symptoms, while others may struggle with several.

Diagnosis:

There isn't a single test for PCOS. Doctors typically diagnose it based on your symptoms and medical history. They may perform the following:

- **Pelvic Exam:** This allows the doctor to check for any abnormalities in your reproductive organs.

- **Blood Tests:** These can measure your hormone levels, including androgens, and check for other conditions like diabetes.
- **Ultrasound:** An ultrasound can help visualize your ovaries and see if they have multiple small cysts, a common feature of PCOS.

Doctors typically diagnose PCOS if you have at least two of the following three criteria:

1. **Irregular Periods**
2. **Signs of Excess Androgen** (either symptoms or blood test results)
3. **Polycystic Ovaries** (seen on ultrasound)

If you're concerned you might have PCOS, talking to your doctor is crucial. Early diagnosis and treatment can help manage symptoms and reduce the risk of long-term complications like diabetes and heart disease.

Role of Diet and Lifestyle in PCOS Management

While PCOS is a hormonal imbalance, the good news is that diet and lifestyle modifications can significantly improve your quality of life and manage many of the symptoms. Here's a detailed breakdown of how these factors play a role:

Diet:

- **Focus on Blood Sugar Control:** PCOS is often linked to insulin resistance, where your body struggles to use insulin effectively. This can lead to blood sugar spikes and crashes. By focusing on foods that don't cause blood sugar spikes, you can help regulate insulin levels and improve overall health.

- **Prioritize Low-Glycemic Index (GI) foods:** The glycemic index (GI) ranks foods based on how quickly they raise blood sugar. Choose low-GI options like whole grains, vegetables, legumes, and lean protein. Limit high-GI foods like white bread, sugary drinks, and processed snacks.
- **Fiber is your friend:** Fiber slows down digestion and helps regulate blood sugar. Aim for plenty of fruits, vegetables, and whole grains in your diet.

- **Manage Inflammation:** Chronic inflammation is linked to many PCOS symptoms. Focus on anti-inflammatory foods like fruits, vegetables, fatty fish (rich in omega-3 fatty acids), and healthy fats (olive oil, nuts, seeds). Limit processed foods, refined carbohydrates, and unhealthy fats (saturated and trans fats) which can promote inflammation.
- **Weight Management:** While not everyone with PCOS is overweight, losing even a moderate amount of weight (5-10%) can significantly improve symptoms like irregular periods and insulin sensitivity.

Lifestyle:

- **Exercise Regularly:** Aim for at least 150 minutes of moderate-intensity exercise per week, or 75 minutes of vigorous exercise. Exercise helps improve insulin sensitivity, manage weight, and reduce inflammation. Even small increases in activity can be beneficial.
- **Prioritize Sleep:** Aim for 7-8 hours of quality sleep each night. Poor sleep can disrupt hormones and worsen PCOS symptoms. Establish a regular sleep schedule and create a relaxing bedtime routine.

- **Manage Stress:** Chronic stress can exacerbate PCOS symptoms. Find healthy ways to manage stress, such as yoga, meditation, deep breathing exercises, or spending time in nature.
- **Consider Supplements:** Some research suggests that certain supplements like inositol, chromium, and omega-3 fatty acids may be helpful for managing PCOS symptoms. **However, it's crucial to talk to your doctor before starting any supplements to ensure they're safe and appropriate for you.**

Remember:

- There's no one-size-fits-all approach. Experiment with different dietary patterns and find what works best for you.
- Consistency is key. Making sustainable changes will have a more significant impact than restrictive fad diets.
- Don't be afraid to seek support. A registered dietitian or PCOS specialist can help you create a personalized plan that addresses your specific needs and goals.

By adopting healthy dietary habits and incorporating a balanced lifestyle, you can take control of your PCOS and live a fulfilling life.

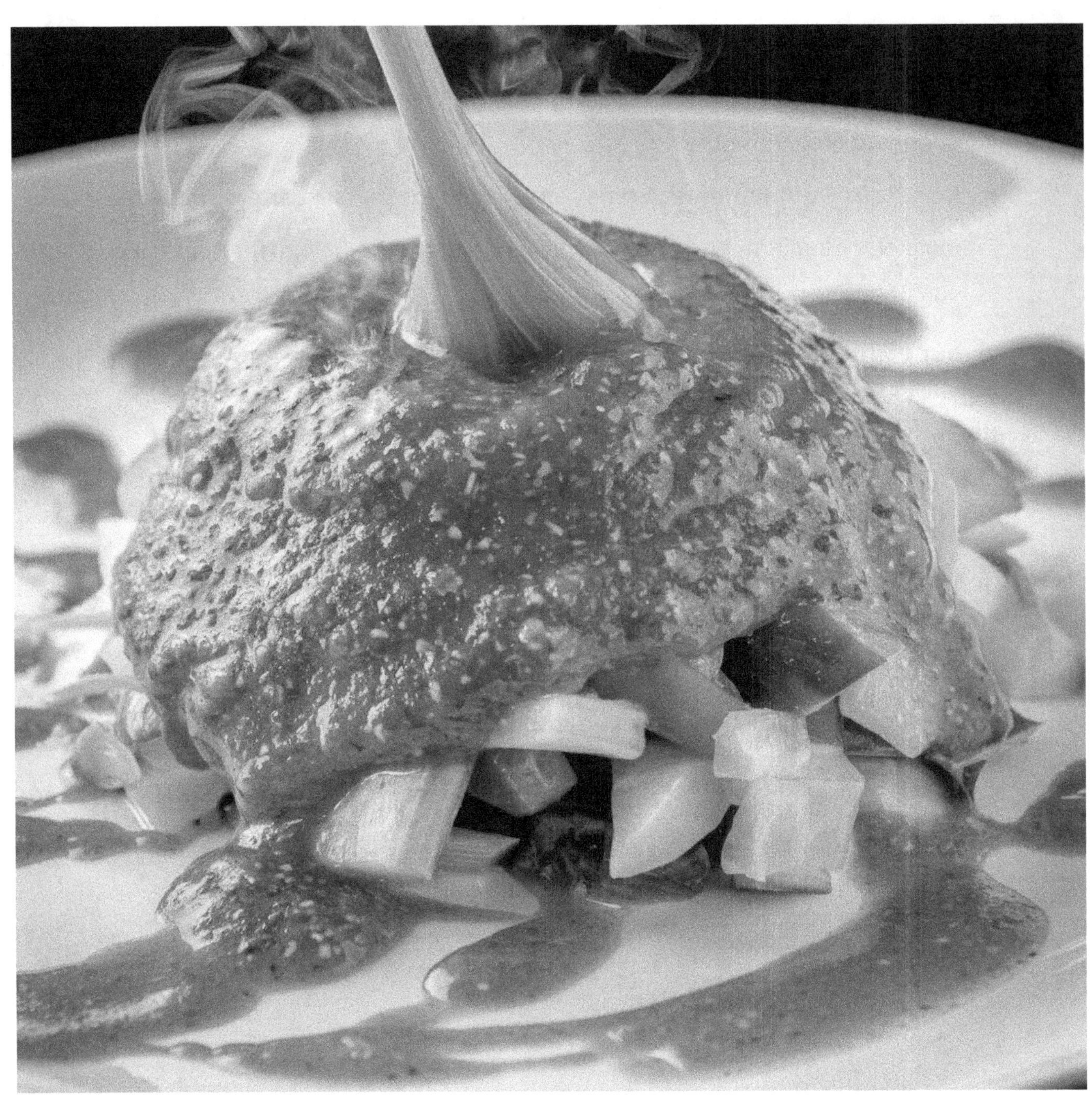

Chapter 2: The PCOS Diet

Key Principles of a PCOS-Friendly Diet

PCOS can feel like a monster lurking in the shadows, but don't despair! A PCOS-friendly diet is a powerful tool to manage symptoms and empower you to take charge of your health. Here are the key principles to keep in mind:

1. Balance Blood Sugar:

- **The Insulin Connection:** With PCOS, your body may struggle to use insulin effectively, leading to blood sugar spikes and crashes. This can worsen symptoms like fatigue, cravings, and weight gain.
- **Low-Glycemic Index (GI) is your Ally:** The GI ranks foods based on how quickly they raise blood sugar. Focus on low-GI options like:
    - **Whole Grains:** Brown rice, quinoa, oats, whole-wheat bread
    - **Vegetables:** Leafy greens, broccoli, carrots, sweet potatoes (with skin)
    - **Legumes:** Beans, lentils, chickpeas
    - **Lean Protein:** Chicken, fish, tofu, tempeh

2. Embrace Fiber:

- **Fiber's Slow and Steady Magic:** Fiber slows down digestion, keeping you feeling fuller for longer and preventing blood sugar spikes. It's a superhero for PCOS management!
- **Fiber-Rich Friends:** Load up your plate with:
    - **Fruits:** Berries, apples, pears, oranges
    - **Vegetables:** All the good stuff mentioned above!
    - **Whole Grains:** See low-GI options

- ○ **Legumes:** Don't forget these powerhouses

3. Fight Inflammation with Food:

- **Chronic inflammation** is linked to many PCOS symptoms. Certain foods can help reduce inflammation:
    - ○ **Antioxidant Powerhouses:** Colorful fruits and vegetables are packed with antioxidants that fight inflammation. Think berries, leafy greens, and peppers.
    - ○ **Omega-3 Rich Fish:** Salmon, tuna, sardines are excellent sources of omega-3 fatty acids with anti-inflammatory properties. Aim for 2 servings per week.
    - ○ **Healthy Fats:** Olive oil, avocado, nuts, and seeds provide healthy fats that can help combat inflammation.

4. Limit Inflammatory Foods:

- **Just Say No to Processed Foods:** Processed foods, refined carbohydrates (white bread, pastries), sugary drinks, and unhealthy fats (saturated and trans fats) can promote inflammation. Minimize these in your diet.

5. Portion Control is Key:

- **Mindful Eating Matters:** While some dietary patterns may work wonders, portion control is crucial for managing weight and overall health. Pay attention to serving sizes and avoid overeating, even healthy foods.

Remember:

- **Individuality Matters:** There's no single "best" PCOS diet. Experiment with different approaches and find what works best for you.

- **Consistency is King:** Making small, sustainable changes will yield better results than restrictive fad diets. Consistency is key!
- **Seek Support:** A registered dietitian or PCOS specialist can be your guide. They can create a personalized plan that addresses your specific needs and goals.

By embracing these key principles, you can transform your diet into a powerful weapon against PCOS. Food becomes your ally, helping you manage symptoms and live a healthy, fulfilling life!

Building Balanced Meals and Snacks

Conquering PCOS often starts on your plate. But with all the information out there, building balanced meals and snacks can feel overwhelming. Here's how to create a PCOS-friendly approach that keeps you satisfied and fights cravings:

The Plate Method:

Imagine your plate divided into sections. Here's what to fill each section with:

- **Half Your Plate: Non-Starchy Vegetables:** These are your low-GI, fiber-rich champions! Load up on leafy greens (spinach, kale), broccoli, cauliflower, peppers, mushrooms, etc. They provide essential nutrients and keep you feeling full.

- **Quarter Your Plate: Lean Protein:** Protein helps regulate blood sugar and keeps you feeling satisfied. Choose lean options like grilled chicken, fish (salmon, tuna), tofu, tempeh, or beans.
- **Quarter Your Plate: Starchy Vegetables or Whole Grains:** Include a source of complex carbohydrates for sustained energy. Brown rice, quinoa, sweet potatoes (with skin!), whole-wheat bread/pasta are great choices. **Be mindful of portion sizes** and opt for whole grains whenever possible.

Don't Forget the Healthy Fats:

Healthy fats are essential for hormone balance and satiety. Include a small portion of healthy fats with each meal:

- **Olive oil:** Drizzle on vegetables or use for cooking.
- **Avocado:** Slice it on salads or toast.
- **Nuts and seeds:** A handful of almonds, walnuts, or chia seeds adds healthy fats and crunch.

Snacking Smart:

Cravings can wreak havoc on your PCOS journey. Here's how to stay ahead of the game:

- **Plan Ahead:** Don't wait until you're starving! Have healthy snacks readily available.
- **Pair Protein and Fiber:** This combo keeps you feeling full for longer. Think apple slices with almond butter, veggie sticks with hummus, or Greek yogurt with berries.
- **Limit Processed Snacks:** Avoid sugary treats, chips, and processed foods. These can trigger blood sugar spikes and cravings.

- **Hydration is Key:** Sometimes thirst can be mistaken for hunger. Drink plenty of water throughout the day to stay hydrated and curb cravings.

Sample Meals and Snacks:

- **Breakfast:** Scrambled eggs with spinach and whole-wheat toast with avocado slices.
- **Snack:** Greek yogurt with berries and a sprinkle of chia seeds.
- **Lunch:** Grilled chicken salad with mixed greens, quinoa, and a light olive oil dressing.
- **Snack:** Carrot sticks with hummus.
- **Dinner:** Salmon with roasted Brussels sprouts and brown rice.

Remember:

- **Variety is Key:** Don't get stuck in a rut! Explore different healthy recipes to keep things interesting.
- **Make it Fun:** Experiment with spices and herbs to add flavor to your meals.
- **Read Food Labels:** Be mindful of hidden sugars and processed ingredients in packaged foods.
- **Listen to Your Body:** Pay attention to how you feel after eating certain foods. Adjust your choices based on what works best for you.

By following these tips and using the plate method as a guide, you can build balanced meals and snacks that fight cravings, keep you satisfied, and support your PCOS management journey. Remember, consistency is key! The more you practice these principles, the easier it becomes to create a PCOS-friendly eating pattern that empowers you to take control of your health.

Tips for Meal Planning and Preparation

Managing PCOS often feels like a juggling act. Between work, family, and other commitments, carving out time for healthy meals can be a challenge. But fear not! Meal planning and preparation can be your secret weapon, saving you time, reducing stress, and ensuring you have delicious, PCOS-friendly options readily available.

Here are some detailed tips to get you started:

Planning Like a Pro:

- **Start Small:** Don't overwhelm yourself! Begin by planning meals for 2-3 days a week. As you get comfortable, you can extend the planning window.
- **Gather Inspiration:** Browse cookbooks, websites, or social media for PCOS-friendly recipes. Consider following registered dietitians or PCOS-specific accounts for reliable information.
- **Consider Your Week:** Think about your schedule and activities. Plan quick and easy meals for busy days and more elaborate options for weekends.
- **Make a List:** Create a grocery list based on your chosen recipes. Include staples you already have on hand to minimize waste.
- **Utilize Apps and Tools:** There are many meal planning apps and online tools that can help you create shopping lists, store recipes, and even generate meal plans based on dietary needs.

Prepping for Success:

- **Set Aside Time:** Dedicate a block of time, like a couple of hours on the weekend, to prepping ingredients. Wash and chop vegetables, cook grains in bulk, portion out protein sources like grilled chicken or tofu.

- **Batch Cooking:** Cook larger portions of certain dishes (soups, stews, lentil curries) that can be used for multiple meals throughout the week. Leftovers become your best friend!
- **Portion Control is Key:** Pre-portioning your meals and snacks into containers helps with portion control and prevents overeating. It's also incredibly convenient for grabbing a quick, healthy meal on the go.
- **Storage Savvy:** Invest in good quality, airtight containers for storing prepped ingredients and meals. Label everything with the date to avoid confusion. Utilize your freezer for longer-term storage of cooked meals or prepped ingredients.

Bonus Tips:

- **Involve the Family:** If possible, get your family involved in meal planning and preparation. It can be a fun bonding activity and teaches valuable life skills.
- **Get Creative with Leftovers:** Don't just reheat leftovers! Leftover cooked chicken can be used in salads, stir-fries, or wraps. Leftover roasted vegetables can be added to omelets or soups.
- **Don't Be Afraid to Adapt:** Recipes are a guide, not a rule book. Feel free to modify recipes to suit your preferences or dietary needs.
- **Be Flexible:** Life happens! If your plans change, don't stress. Frozen vegetables are a great option to have on hand for quick, healthy sides.

Remember:

- **Consistency is Key:** The more you practice meal planning and preparation, the easier it becomes. Start small and build a routine that works for you.
- **Enjoy the Process:** Cooking can be a fun and creative way to nourish your body. Experiment with new flavors and recipes to keep things interesting.

- **Celebrate Your Wins:** Meal planning and preparation take effort. Acknowledge your progress and celebrate the time you're saving and the healthy choices you're making!

By following these tips, you can transform meal planning and preparation into a powerful tool for managing your PCOS. It will save you time, reduce stress, and ensure you have delicious, nutritious meals readily available, empowering you to live a healthy and fulfilling life.

Chapter 3: Recipes Makeup Meals

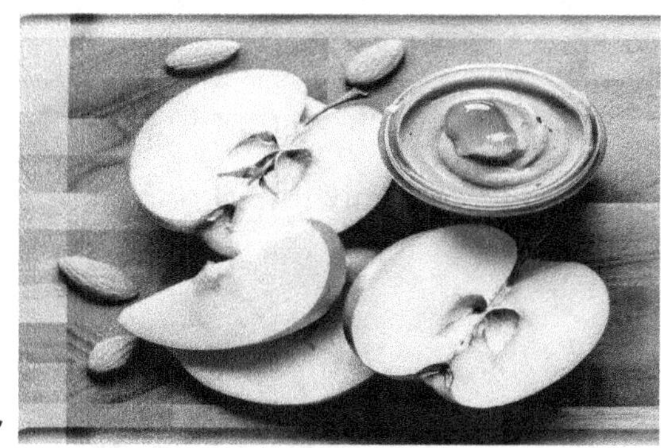

Apple slices with almond butter

This is the simplest version and requires no cooking:

- Ingredients:
    1. 1 apple (your favorite variety)
    2. 2 tablespoons almond butter (smooth or crunchy, depending on your preference)
- Instructions:
    1. Wash and dry your apple.
    2. Slice the apple into thin or thick slices, depending on your preference.
    3. Spread almond butter on each apple slice.
    4. Enjoy!

Spiced Apple Slices with Almond Butter:

This recipe adds a touch of warmth and flavor with cinnamon.

- Ingredients:
    1. 1 apple (your favorite variety)
    2. 2 tablespoons almond butter (smooth or crunchy, depending on your preference)
    3. 1/4 teaspoon ground cinnamon

4. Pinch of nutmeg (optional)

- Instructions:

    1. Wash and dry your apple.

    2. Slice the apple into thin or thick slices, depending on your preference.

    3. In a small bowl, mix the almond butter with the cinnamon and nutmeg (if using).

    4. Spread the spiced almond butter on each apple slice.

    5. Enjoy!

Chocolate Drizzled Apple Slices with Almond Butter:

This recipe adds a touch of sweetness with melted chocolate.

- Ingredients:

    1. 1 apple (your favorite variety)

    2. 2 tablespoons almond butter (smooth or crunchy, depending on your preference)

    3. 1 ounce dark chocolate (chopped or chips)

    4. 1 teaspoon coconut oil (optional)

- Instructions:

    1. Wash and dry your apple.

    2. Slice the apple into thin or thick slices, depending on your preference.

    3. Spread almond butter on each apple slice.

    4. In a small heatproof bowl, melt the chocolate with the coconut oil (if using) over a double boiler or in the microwave on low power, stirring frequently.

    5. Once melted, drizzle the chocolate over the apple slices with almond butter.

    6. Let the chocolate cool and harden slightly before enjoying.

Extra Tips:

- For a more decadent treat, sprinkle the chocolate with chopped nuts, shredded coconut, or a pinch of sea salt before it hardens.
- If you don't have any almond butter, other nut butters like peanut butter or cashew butter can be used as a substitute.
- To prevent apple slices from browning, you can toss them in a little lemon juice after slicing.
- These apple slices with almond butter can be stored in an airtight container in the refrigerator for up to 2 days. However, the apple slices may brown slightly.

Carrot sticks with hummus

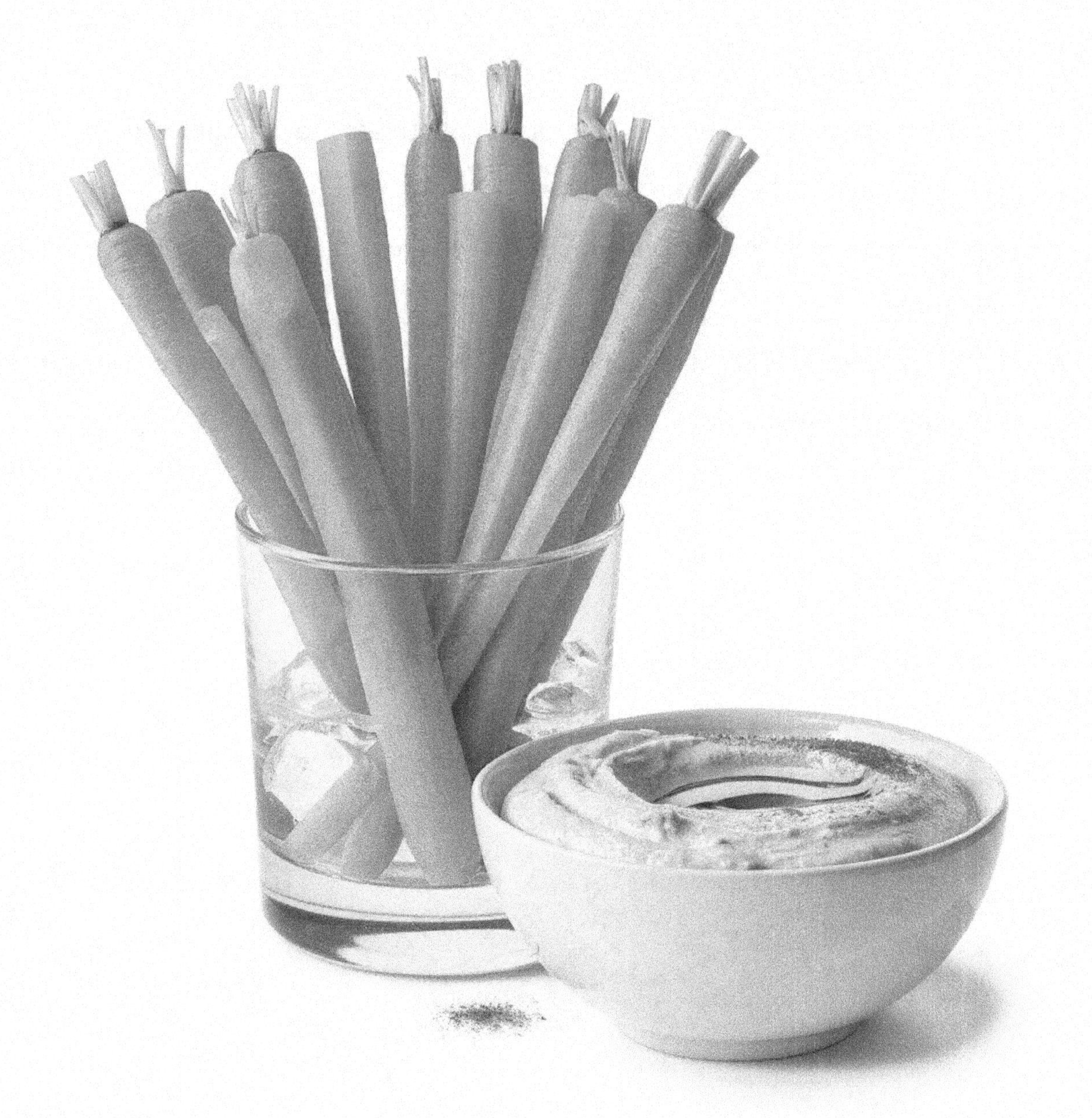

Ingredients:

1. Carrots (washed and cut into sticks)
2. Hummus (store-bought or homemade - see below for a basic recipe)

- Instructions:
    1. Wash and dry your carrots.
    2. Cut the carrots into sticks of your desired thickness.
    3. Serve the carrot sticks with your favorite hummus.

Spiced Carrot Sticks with Hummus and Yogurt Dip:

This recipe adds a tangy and flavorful twist with a yogurt dip.

- Ingredients:
    1. Carrots (washed and cut into sticks)
    2. Hummus (store-bought or homemade)
    3. For the Yogurt Dip:
        - 1/2 cup plain Greek yogurt
        - 1 tablespoon lemon juice
        - 1/4 teaspoon ground cumin
        - Pinch of salt and pepper
- Instructions:
    1. Prepare the carrots as in the classic recipe.
    2. For the yogurt dip, whisk together the Greek yogurt, lemon juice, cumin, salt, and pepper in a small bowl.
    3. Serve the carrot sticks with both hummus and the yogurt dip for a variety of flavors.

Roasted Carrot Sticks with Herb Hummus:

This recipe adds a roasted and flavorful twist to the carrots and uses a simple herb hummus variation.

- Ingredients:
    1. Carrots (washed and cut into sticks)
    2. Olive oil
    3. Salt and pepper
    4. For the Herb Hummus:
        - 1 can (15 oz) chickpeas, drained and rinsed
        - 2 tablespoons tahini
        - 2 tablespoons olive oil
        - 1/4 cup lemon juice
        - 1 clove garlic, minced
        - 1/4 cup fresh parsley, chopped
        - 1/4 cup fresh cilantro, chopped
        - Salt and pepper to taste
- Instructions:
    1. Preheat the oven to 400°F (200°C).
    2. Toss carrot sticks with olive oil, salt, and pepper. Spread them on a baking sheet and roast for 15-20 minutes, or until tender-crisp.
    3. For the herb hummus, combine all ingredients in a food processor and blend until smooth.
    4. Serve the roasted carrot sticks with the herb hummus.

Extra Tips:

- You can experiment with different types of hummus flavors like roasted red pepper, roasted garlic, or olive tapenade.

- For added crunch, sprinkle the carrot sticks with everything bagel seasoning or sesame seeds before or after roasting.
- Store leftover carrot sticks in an airtight container in the refrigerator for up to 3 days. Hummus can be stored in the refrigerator for up to a week.

Greek yogurt with berries

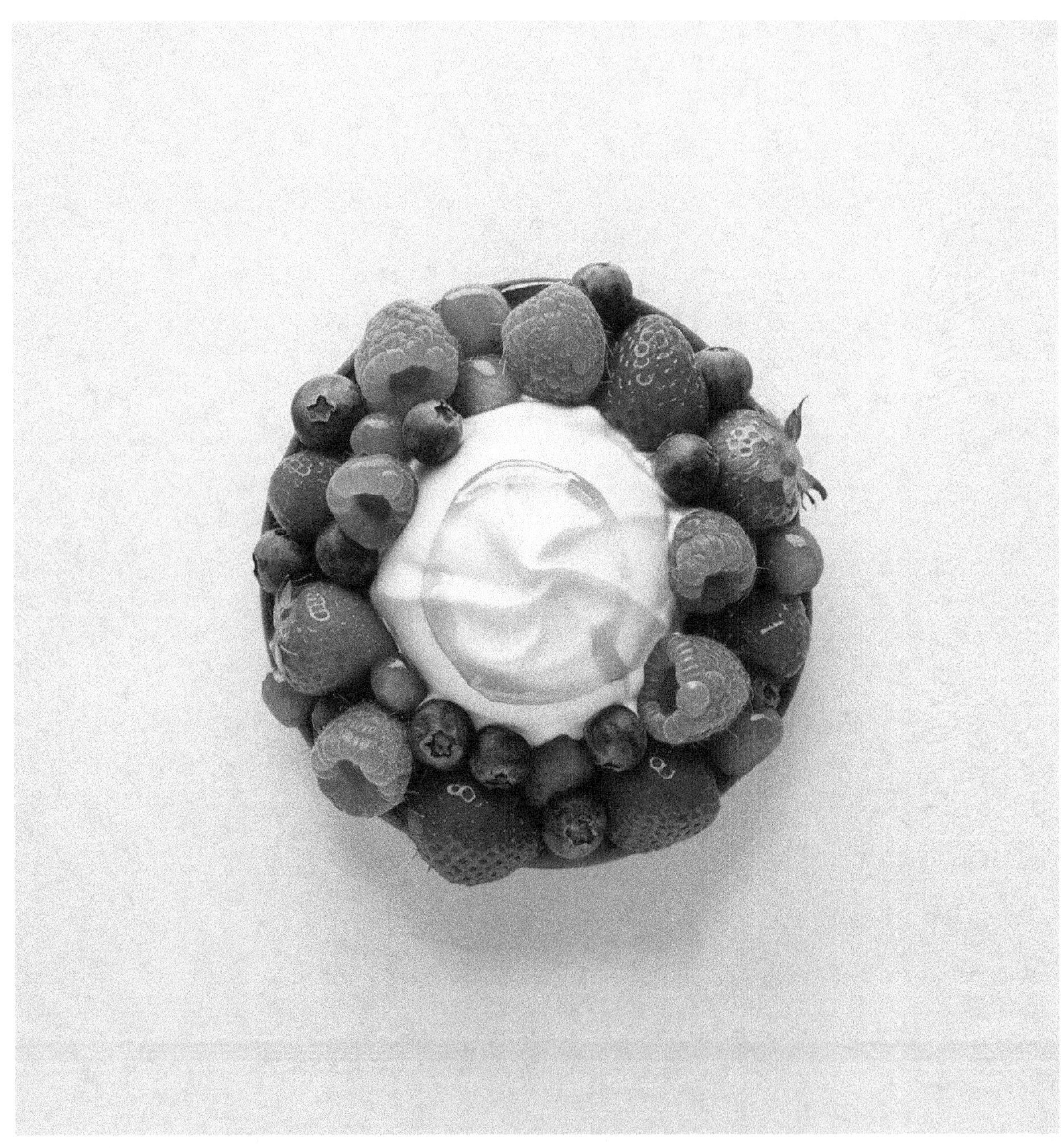

Ingredients:

1. 1 cup plain Greek yogurt (2% or non-fat)
2. 1/2 cup fresh berries (your favorites like blueberries, strawberries, raspberries, blackberries)
3. 1 tablespoon honey or maple syrup (optional)
4. Granola or chopped nuts (optional)

- Instructions:

1. In a bowl, spoon in your Greek yogurt.
2. Wash and dry your berries. Add them to the yogurt.
3. Drizzle with honey or maple syrup for extra sweetness (optional).
4. Sprinkle with granola or chopped nuts for added texture and crunch (optional).
5. Enjoy!

Layered Greek Yogurt Parfait with Berries:

This version creates a visually appealing and layered parfait.

- Ingredients:

1. 1 cup plain Greek yogurt (2% or non-fat)
2. 1/2 cup fresh berries (your favorites)
3. 1/4 cup granola (optional)
4. Chia seeds (optional)
5. Fresh mint leaves (optional)

- Instructions:

1. In a clear glass or jar, layer the ingredients in this order:
   - Greek yogurt
   - Berries

    ■ Granola (if using)

    ■ Repeat layers (optional)

2. Top with chia seeds and fresh mint leaves for a finishing touch (optional).

3. Enjoy!

Protein-Packed Greek Yogurt Bowl with Berries and Granola:

This recipe adds a protein boost with protein powder and provides a more substantial snack or breakfast.

- Ingredients:
    1. 1 cup plain Greek yogurt (2% or non-fat)
    2. 1/2 cup fresh berries (your favorites)
    3. 1/4 cup granola
    4. 1 scoop protein powder (unflavored or vanilla preferred)
    5. 1/4 cup almond milk (optional)
- Instructions:
    1. In a bowl, combine the Greek yogurt and protein powder. If the mixture seems too thick, add a splash of almond milk to thin it out.
    2. Wash and dry your berries. Add them to the yogurt mixture.
    3. Top with granola for added texture and crunch.
    4. Enjoy!

Extra Tips:

- You can experiment with different types of berries or add other fruits like chopped banana, mango, or peaches.
- For a frozen yogurt treat, freeze individual portions of Greek yogurt with berries in airtight containers for a few hours.

- You can use flavored Greek yogurt varieties like vanilla or honey, but be mindful of added sugar content.
- Consider adding a sprinkle of cinnamon or a drizzle of nut butter for extra flavor variations.

Handful of nuts and seeds

A handful of nuts and seeds is a fantastic PCOS-friendly snack, but it doesn't need a recipe! However, there are ways to enjoy them with a bit more variety and flavor. Here are some ideas:

Spiced Nut and Seed Mix:

- Combine a handful of raw or roasted nuts and seeds of your choice (almonds, walnuts, cashews, pumpkin seeds, sunflower seeds, chia seeds, flaxseeds).
- In a small bowl, toss them with a sprinkle of your favorite spices like cinnamon, chili powder, curry powder, or everything bagel seasoning.
- You can also add a touch of olive oil or melted coconut oil for extra flavor and to help the spices adhere.

Trail Mix Variation:

- Combine your favorite nuts and seeds with dried fruits like cranberries, raisins, or chopped dates for a sweet and salty mix.
- You can also add some dark chocolate chips or granola for extra texture and flavor.

- Be mindful of portion control with dried fruits, as they are higher in sugar than nuts and seeds.

Yogurt Topping:

- Add a handful of chopped nuts and seeds to your favorite Greek yogurt or oatmeal for extra protein, healthy fats, and a satisfying crunch.

Salad Topping:

- Sprinkle a handful of nuts and seeds over your salad for added texture, flavor, and a nutritional boost.
- This works well with various salads, from classic green salads to heartier options with quinoa or brown rice.

Energy Bites (No-Bake Option):

- Combine nuts, seeds, dried fruits (optional), rolled oats, and a natural binding agent like honey, nut butter, or mashed dates.
- Form small balls and refrigerate for a healthy and satisfying snack on the go.

Remember:

- Be mindful of portion sizes. A handful is generally considered 1 ounce or about 2 tablespoons.
- Opt for unsalted or dry-roasted nuts and seeds whenever possible to limit sodium intake.
- Choose raw or minimally processed nuts and seeds for the most health benefits.

Enjoy your handful of nuts and seeds with a touch of creativity!

Cottage cheese with chopped vegetables

Cottage cheese with chopped vegetables is a delicious and nutritious PCOS-friendly snack or light meal. Here are some recipe ideas to take it beyond the basics:

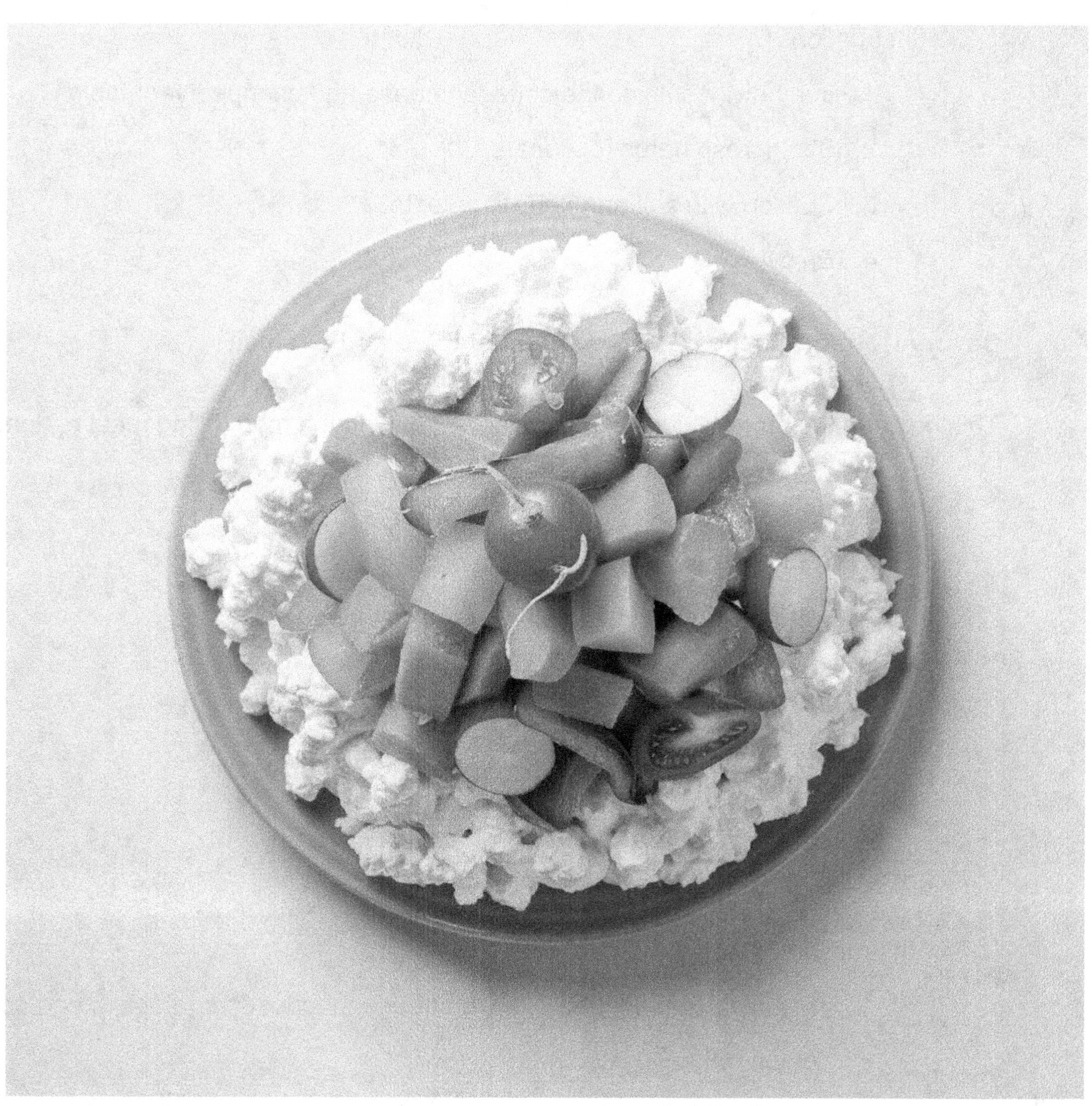

Ingredients:

1. 1/2 cup cottage cheese (low-fat or 2%)
2. 1/2 cup chopped vegetables (your favorites like cucumber, tomatoes, bell peppers, red onion)
3. Fresh herbs (optional: chopped parsley, dill, chives)
4. Salt and pepper to taste

- Instructions:

1. In a bowl, combine the cottage cheese and chopped vegetables.
2. Stir in fresh herbs (optional).
3. Season with salt and pepper to taste.
4. Enjoy!

Savory Cottage Cheese Salad with Vegetables and Grains:

This recipe adds more texture and substance, making it a more filling meal option.

- Ingredients:

1. 1 cup cottage cheese (low-fat or 2%)
2. 1/2 cup chopped vegetables (your favorites)
3. 1/4 cup cooked quinoa or brown rice
4. Kalamata olives (optional, sliced)
5. Extra virgin olive oil (optional)
6. Lemon juice (optional)
7. Salt and pepper to taste

- Instructions:

1. In a bowl, combine the cottage cheese, chopped vegetables, and cooked quinoa or brown rice.
2. Add sliced Kalamata olives for a salty and briny flavor (optional).

3. Drizzle with a touch of olive oil and lemon juice for extra flavor (optional).

4. Season with salt and pepper to taste.

5. Enjoy!

Spicy Cottage Cheese Dip with Veggie Sticks:

This recipe transforms cottage cheese into a delicious dip perfect for crudités.

- Ingredients:
  1. 1 cup cottage cheese (low-fat or 2%)
  2. 1/4 cup chopped vegetables (roasted red peppers, sun-dried tomatoes)
  3. 1-2 tablespoons finely chopped fresh herbs (cilantro, chives)
  4. 1/4 teaspoon chili powder (adjust to your spice preference)
  5. Pinch of smoked paprika (optional)
  6. Salt and pepper to taste
  7. Vegetable sticks (celery, carrots, bell peppers) for dipping
- Instructions:
  1. In a food processor or blender, combine the cottage cheese, chopped vegetables, herbs, chili powder, smoked paprika (optional), salt, and pepper.
  2. Blend until smooth, but be careful not to over-blend. You want a slightly chunky consistency.
  3. Serve the cottage cheese dip with your favorite vegetable sticks for dipping.

Extra Tips:

- Experiment with different vegetable combinations. Chopped broccoli, zucchini, or mushrooms can be great additions.

- For a protein boost, add some chopped cooked shrimp, grilled chicken, or crumbled tofu.
- Serve cottage cheese with chopped fruit like pineapple, mango, or berries for a sweet and savory twist.
- Leftovers can be stored in an airtight container in the refrigerator for up to 2 days.

Enjoy your cottage cheese with chopped vegetables and explore different flavor combinations to keep it interesting!

Hard-boiled egg

Hard-boiled eggs are a versatile and protein-packed PCOS-friendly food. They can be enjoyed on their own as a snack or incorporated into various recipes. Here are some recipe ideas to elevate your hard-boiled egg game:

Classic Deviled Eggs:

- This timeless appetizer is always a crowd-pleaser.
- You can find countless variations online, but here's a basic recipe: Ingredients: * 6 hard-boiled eggs * 1/4 cup mayonnaise * 1 tablespoon mustard (Dijon or yellow) * Salt and pepper to taste * Paprika (optional, for garnish) Instructions: 1. Peel the hard-boiled eggs and carefully cut them in half lengthwise. 2. Remove the yolks and mash them in a bowl with mayonnaise, mustard, salt, and pepper. 3. You can add other ingredients to the yolk mixture like chopped herbs, crumbled cheese, or a touch of hot sauce for a flavor twist. 4.

Spoon the yolk mixture back into the egg whites. 5. Garnish with paprika (optional) and serve.

Simple Egg Salad:

- This is a great option for sandwiches, wraps, or a light salad on its own.
  Ingredients: * 4 hard-boiled eggs, chopped * 2 tablespoons mayonnaise (or plain Greek yogurt for a lighter option) * 1 tablespoon chopped celery (optional) * 1 tablespoon chopped red onion (optional) * Chopped fresh herbs (optional: parsley, chives) * Salt and pepper to taste
  Instructions: 1. In a bowl, combine the chopped hard-boiled eggs, mayonnaise or yogurt, celery (optional), red onion (optional), and fresh herbs (optional). 2. Season with salt and pepper to taste. 3. Serve on bread as a sandwich filling, in a wrap, or with lettuce leaves for a salad.

Egg and Avocado Toast:

- This is a trendy and satisfying breakfast or snack option.
  Ingredients: * 1 slice whole-wheat toast * 1/2 ripe avocado, mashed * 1 hard-boiled egg, sliced * Salt and pepper to taste * Hot sauce (optional)
  Instructions: 1. Toast your whole-wheat bread slice. 2. Spread mashed avocado on the toast. 3. Top with sliced hard-boiled egg. 4. Season with salt, pepper, and hot sauce (optional) to taste.

Cobb Salad with Hard-Boiled Egg:

- This classic salad gets a protein boost with hard-boiled eggs.
  Ingredients: * Mixed greens * Grilled chicken breast, sliced * Avocado, diced * crumbled blue cheese * Cherry tomatoes, halved * 1 hard-boiled egg, sliced * Vinaigrette dressing

Instructions: 1. In a large bowl, combine mixed greens, grilled chicken slices, avocado, blue cheese, cherry tomatoes, and sliced hard-boiled egg. 2. Drizzle with your favorite vinaigrette dressing and toss to coat.

Bonus Tip:

- Hard-boiled eggs are also a great addition to ramen bowls, soups, and grain salads. They add protein and a delightful textural contrast.

Remember:

- You can adjust these recipes to your taste preferences. Experiment with different ingredients and flavors.
- Prepping a batch of hard-boiled eggs at the beginning of the week makes it easier to incorporate them into your meals and snacks throughout the week.

Snack Sides and Appetizers

Mini lentil or black bean burgers

Here are two delicious recipes for mini lentil or black bean burgers, perfect for PCOS-friendly snacks or light meals:

Spiced Lentil Burgers:

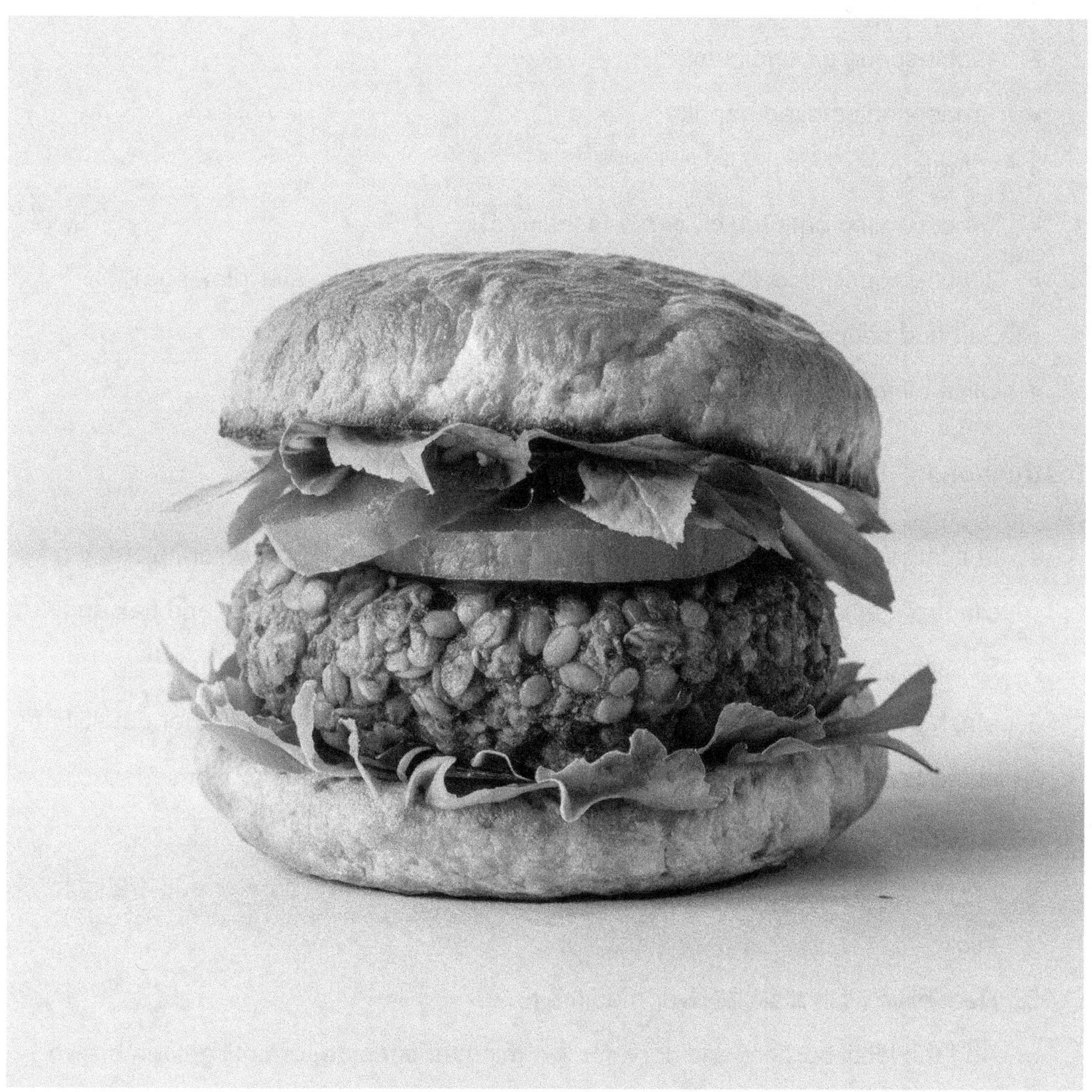

Ingredients:

- 1 cup cooked brown lentils
- 1/2 cup cooked quinoa (optional, for added texture)
- 1/2 cup finely chopped red onion
- 1/4 cup chopped fresh parsley

- 1/4 cup chopped cilantro
- 1 clove garlic, minced
- 1 tablespoon ground cumin
- 1 teaspoon smoked paprika
- 1/2 teaspoon chili powder
- 1/4 cup rolled oats (quick or old-fashioned)
- 2 tablespoons flaxseed meal mixed with 6 tablespoons water (flax egg)
- Salt and pepper to taste
- Olive oil for cooking

Instructions:

1. In a large bowl, combine cooked lentils, quinoa (if using), red onion, parsley, cilantro, garlic, cumin, smoked paprika, chili powder, rolled oats, and flax egg.
2. Season generously with salt and pepper.
3. Mash the mixture with a fork or potato masher until it comes together but still has some texture. You can also use a food processor with pulse motions for a smoother consistency.
4. Form the mixture into small patties, about 2-3 inches in diameter and 1/2 inch thick.
5. Heat olive oil in a skillet over medium heat.
6. Add the lentil burgers and cook for 3-4 minutes per side, or until golden brown and heated through.
7. Serve on whole-wheat buns with your favorite toppings like lettuce, tomato, sliced avocado, and a light yogurt sauce.

Black Bean Burgers with Chipotle Mayo:

Ingredients:

- 1 can (15 oz) black beans, drained and rinsed
- 1/2 cup cooked brown rice
- 1/4 cup chopped red bell pepper
- 1/4 cup chopped green onion
- 1/4 cup chopped fresh cilantro
- 1 jalapeno pepper, seeded and finely chopped (optional, for a spicy kick)
- 1 tablespoon lime juice
- 1 teaspoon ground cumin
- 1/2 teaspoon chili powder
- 1/4 cup breadcrumbs
- 1 egg (or 1 flax egg for a vegan option)
- Salt and pepper to taste
- Olive oil for cooking

For the Chipotle Mayo:

- 1/2 cup mayonnaise (light or Greek yogurt)
- 1 tablespoon chopped chipotle pepper in adobo sauce (adjust to your spice preference)
- 1 tablespoon lime juice
- Salt and pepper to taste

Instructions:

1. In a large bowl, mash together the black beans with a fork or potato masher. Don't mash them completely; you want some texture.
2. Add cooked brown rice, red bell pepper, green onion, cilantro, jalapeno (if using), lime juice, cumin, chili powder, breadcrumbs, and egg (or flax egg).
3. Season with salt and pepper to taste.

4. Mix well and form the mixture into small patties, about the same size as the lentil burgers.

5. In a small bowl, combine the ingredients for the chipotle mayo.

6. Heat olive oil in a skillet over medium heat.

7. Add the black bean burgers and cook for 3-4 minutes per side, or until golden brown and heated through.

8. Serve on whole-wheat buns with your favorite toppings and a dollop of chipotle mayo.

Tips:

- You can bake the burgers instead of pan-frying them. Preheat the oven to 400°F (200°C). Lightly grease a baking sheet and bake the burgers for 15-20 minutes per side, or until golden brown and heated through.
- Leftover burgers can be stored in an airtight container in the refrigerator for up to 3 days. Reheat in a skillet or microwave until warmed through.
- Feel free to experiment with different spices and herbs to create your own flavor variations.

Enjoy these delicious and healthy mini lentil or black bean burgers!

Cauliflower bites

Cauliflower bites are a delicious and healthy alternative to traditional fried foods. They are perfect for a PCOS-friendly snack, appetizer, or even a side dish. Here are two recipe ideas to get you started:

Classic Crispy Cauliflower Bites:

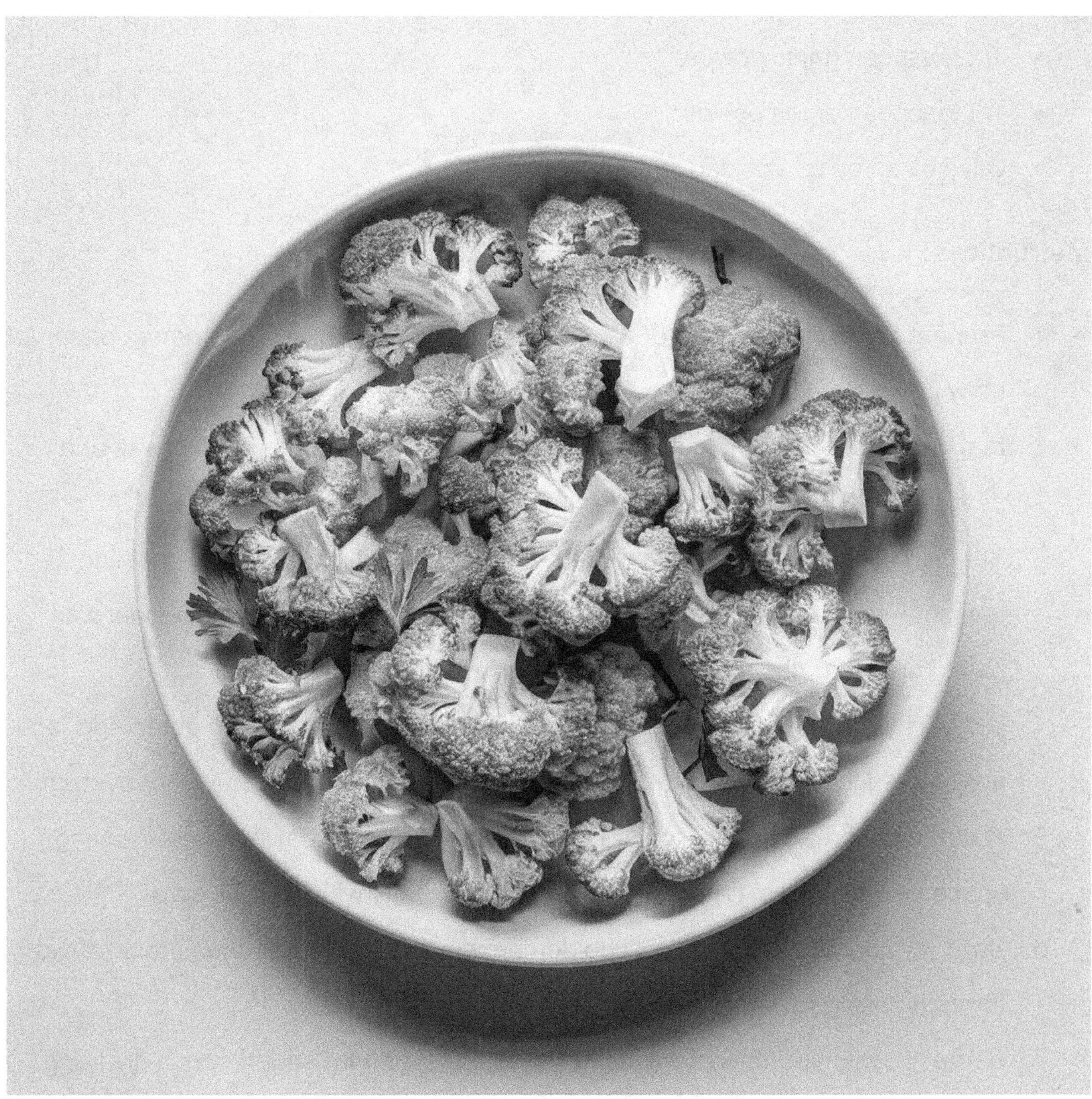

Ingredients:

- 1 head of cauliflower, cut into bite-sized florets
- 1 cup all-purpose flour (or gluten-free alternative)
- 2 large eggs, beaten
- 1 1/3 cups panko breadcrumbs

- 1 1/4 teaspoons fine sea salt, divided
- 1 1/4 teaspoons black pepper, divided
- 1/2 teaspoon garlic powder
- 1/2 teaspoon onion powder
- Olive oil spray for cooking

Instructions:

1. Preheat the oven to 400°F (200°C). Line a baking sheet with parchment paper for easy cleanup.
2. In a large bowl, toss the cauliflower florets with 1/4 teaspoon each of salt and pepper.
3. Set up a breading station with three bowls: one with flour and the remaining 1 teaspoon each of salt and pepper, another with beaten eggs, and the last with panko breadcrumbs mixed with the garlic and onion powder.
4. Dip each cauliflower floret in the flour mixture, then coat it in the beaten egg, and finally, dredge it in the panko breadcrumb mixture, ensuring complete coverage.
5. Arrange the breaded cauliflower florets on the prepared baking sheet, leaving space between them for even cooking. Spray lightly with olive oil spray.
6. Bake for 20-25 minutes, or until golden brown and crispy. Flip the florets halfway through baking for even browning.
7. Serve hot with your favorite dipping sauce like marinara sauce, ranch dressing, or a yogurt-based dip.

Buffalo Cauliflower Bites (Spicy Option):

This recipe adds a spicy kick to the cauliflower bites with a flavorful buffalo sauce coating.

Ingredients:

- 1 head of cauliflower, cut into bite-sized florets
- 1/2 cup all-purpose flour (or gluten-free alternative)
- 2 large eggs, beaten
- 1 1/3 cups panko breadcrumbs
- 1/2 cup hot sauce (adjust to your spice preference)
- 2 tablespoons melted butter
- 1/4 cup chopped fresh parsley (optional, for garnish)
- 1/4 cup crumbled blue cheese (optional, for garnish)
- Olive oil spray for cooking

Instructions:

1. Preheat the oven to 400°F (200°C). Line a baking sheet with parchment paper.
2. In a large bowl, toss the cauliflower florets with a pinch of salt.
3. Set up a breading station similar to the classic recipe: flour, beaten eggs, and panko breadcrumbs.
4. Dip each cauliflower floret in the flour, then coat it in the beaten egg, and finally, dredge it in the panko breadcrumbs.
5. Arrange the breaded cauliflower florets on the prepared baking sheet, leaving space between them. Spray lightly with olive oil spray.
6. Bake for 20-25 minutes, or until golden brown and crispy. Flip the florets halfway through baking.
7. While the cauliflower bakes, in a small bowl, combine the hot sauce and melted butter to create a buffalo sauce.
8. Once the cauliflower bites are cooked, toss them in the buffalo sauce to coat them evenly.

9. Serve hot garnished with chopped fresh parsley and crumbled blue cheese (optional).

Tips:

- For an air-fryer option, preheat your air fryer to 400°F (200°C) and cook the breaded cauliflower florets for 15-20 minutes, shaking the basket occasionally, or until golden brown and crispy.
- You can experiment with different seasonings and spices in the flour mixture to create different flavor variations.
- Leftover cauliflower bites can be stored in an airtight container in the refrigerator for up to 3 days. Reheat in a preheated oven or air fryer until warmed through and crispy again.

Enjoy these delicious and healthy cauliflower bites!

Stuffed mini peppers

Stuffed mini peppers are a versatile and fun appetizer or light meal option, perfect for a PCOS-friendly diet. Here are some recipe ideas to inspire your culinary creations:

Classic Cheesy Sausage Peppers:

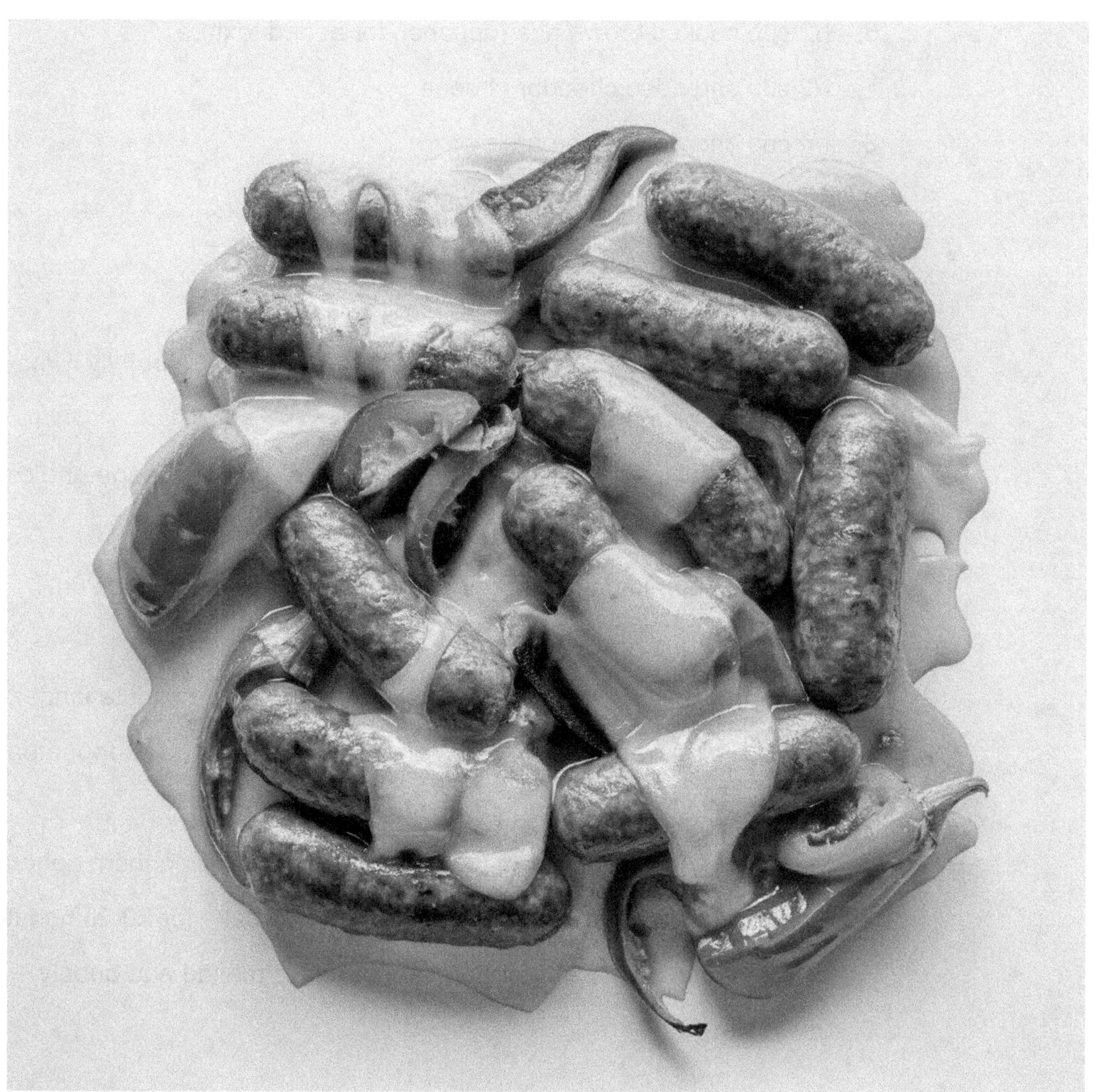

Ingredients:

1. 12 mini bell peppers (assorted colors for visual appeal)

2. 1 tablespoon olive oil

3. 1/2 pound Italian sausage (mild or hot, depending on your preference), casings removed

4. 1/2 cup chopped onion

5. 1/2 cup chopped mushrooms

6. 1/2 cup cooked brown rice (optional, for added texture)

7. 1/2 cup shredded cheddar cheese

8. 1/4 cup chopped fresh parsley

9. Salt and pepper to taste

- Instructions:

1. Preheat the oven to 375°F (190°C).

2. Wash and dry the mini peppers. Cut off the tops and carefully remove the seeds and membranes.

3. Heat olive oil in a skillet over medium heat. Add the sausage and cook until browned, breaking it up with a spoon.

4. Add the chopped onion and mushrooms to the pan and cook until softened.

5. Stir in the cooked brown rice (if using) and cook for a minute longer.

6. Remove from heat and stir in the shredded cheese and chopped parsley. Season with salt and pepper to taste.

7. Stuff the pepper halves with the sausage mixture, filling them generously.

8. Place the stuffed peppers in a baking dish and bake for 20-25 minutes, or until the peppers are tender and the cheese is melted and bubbly.

9. Serve warm.

Vegetarian Quinoa Stuffed Peppers:

This recipe offers a vegetarian twist with a protein-packed quinoa filling:

- Ingredients:

1. 12 mini bell peppers (assorted colors)

2. 1 tablespoon olive oil

3. 1 cup cooked quinoa

4. 1/2 cup chopped onion

5. 1/2 cup chopped bell pepper (another color for a visual contrast)

6. 1/2 cup chopped zucchini

7. 1/4 cup crumbled feta cheese (optional)

8. 1/4 cup chopped fresh parsley

9. 1 tablespoon chopped fresh thyme

10. 1/4 cup vegetable broth

11. Salt and pepper to taste

- Instructions:

1. Preheat the oven to 375°F (190°C).

2. Wash and dry the mini peppers. Cut off the tops and carefully remove the seeds and membranes.

3. Heat olive oil in a skillet over medium heat. Add the chopped onion, bell pepper, and zucchini. Sauté for 5-7 minutes, or until softened.

4. Stir in the cooked quinoa and cook for a minute longer.

5. Remove from heat and stir in the crumbled feta cheese (if using), chopped parsley, and thyme. Season with salt and pepper to taste.

6. Moisten the mixture with the vegetable broth if needed for better consistency.

7. Stuff the pepper halves with the quinoa mixture, filling them generously.

8. Place the stuffed peppers in a baking dish and bake for 20-25 minutes, or until the peppers are tender and the filling is heated through.

9. Serve warm.

Spicy Black Bean and Corn Stuffed Peppers:

This recipe incorporates Mexican flavors with a touch of spice:

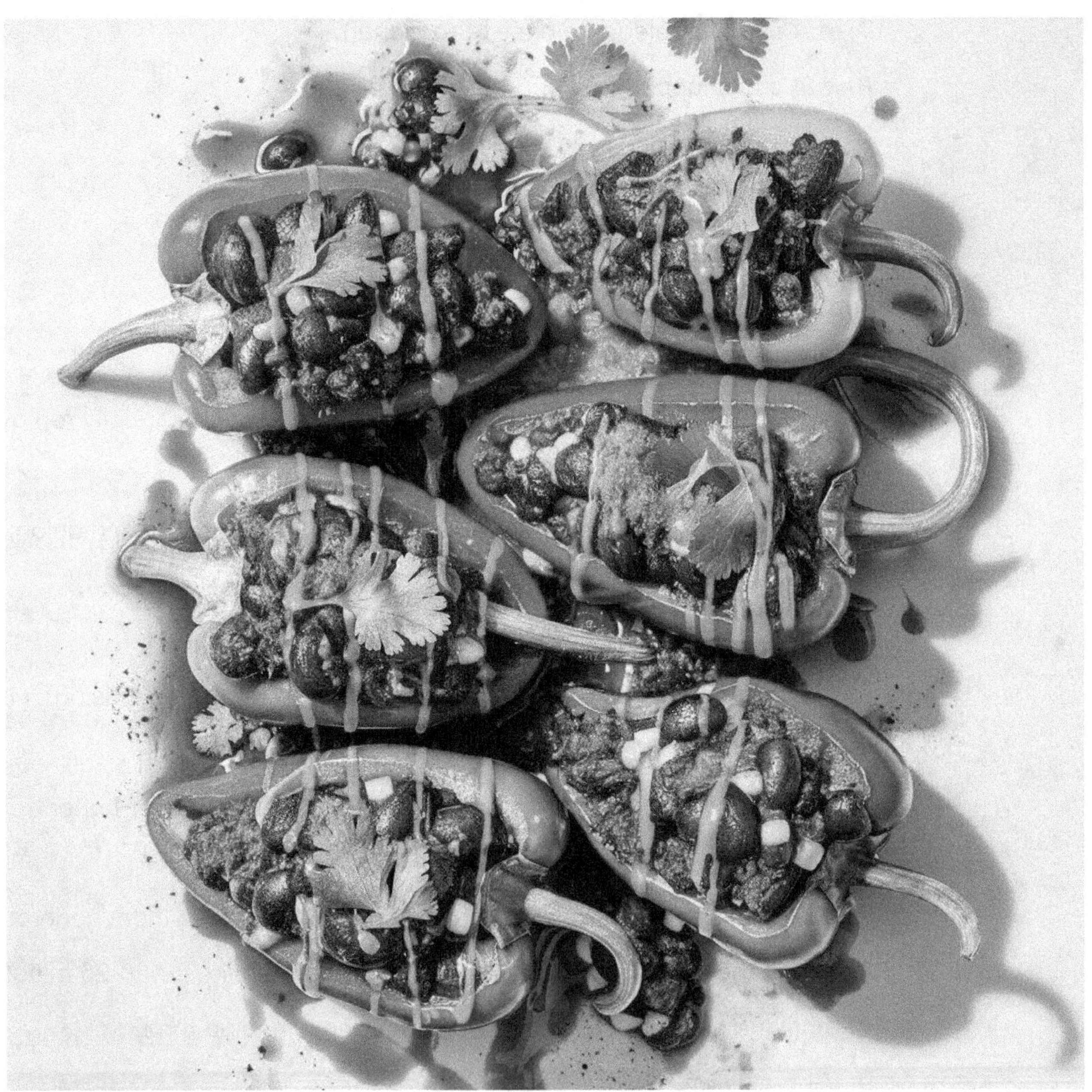

Ingredients:

1. 12 mini bell peppers (assorted colors)

2. 1 tablespoon olive oil

3. 1 can (15 oz) black beans, rinsed and drained

4. 1/2 cup frozen corn, thawed

5. 1/2 cup chopped onion

6. 1/4 cup chopped red bell pepper

7. 1 jalapeno pepper, seeded and finely chopped (adjust to your spice preference)

8. 1/4 cup chopped fresh cilantro

9. 1 tablespoon taco seasoning

10. 1/4 cup shredded Monterey Jack cheese

11. Salt and pepper to taste

- Instructions:

1. Preheat the oven to 375°F (190°C).

2. Wash and dry the mini peppers. Cut off the tops and carefully remove the seeds and membranes.

3. Heat olive oil in a skillet over medium heat. Add the chopped onion, red bell pepper, and jalapeno (if using). Sauté for 5 minutes, or until softened.

4. Stir in the black beans, corn, and taco seasoning. Cook for another minute, stirring to coat the beans and corn in the seasoning.

5. Remove from heat and stir in the chopped cilantro and shredded Monterey Jack cheese

Vegetable spring rolls

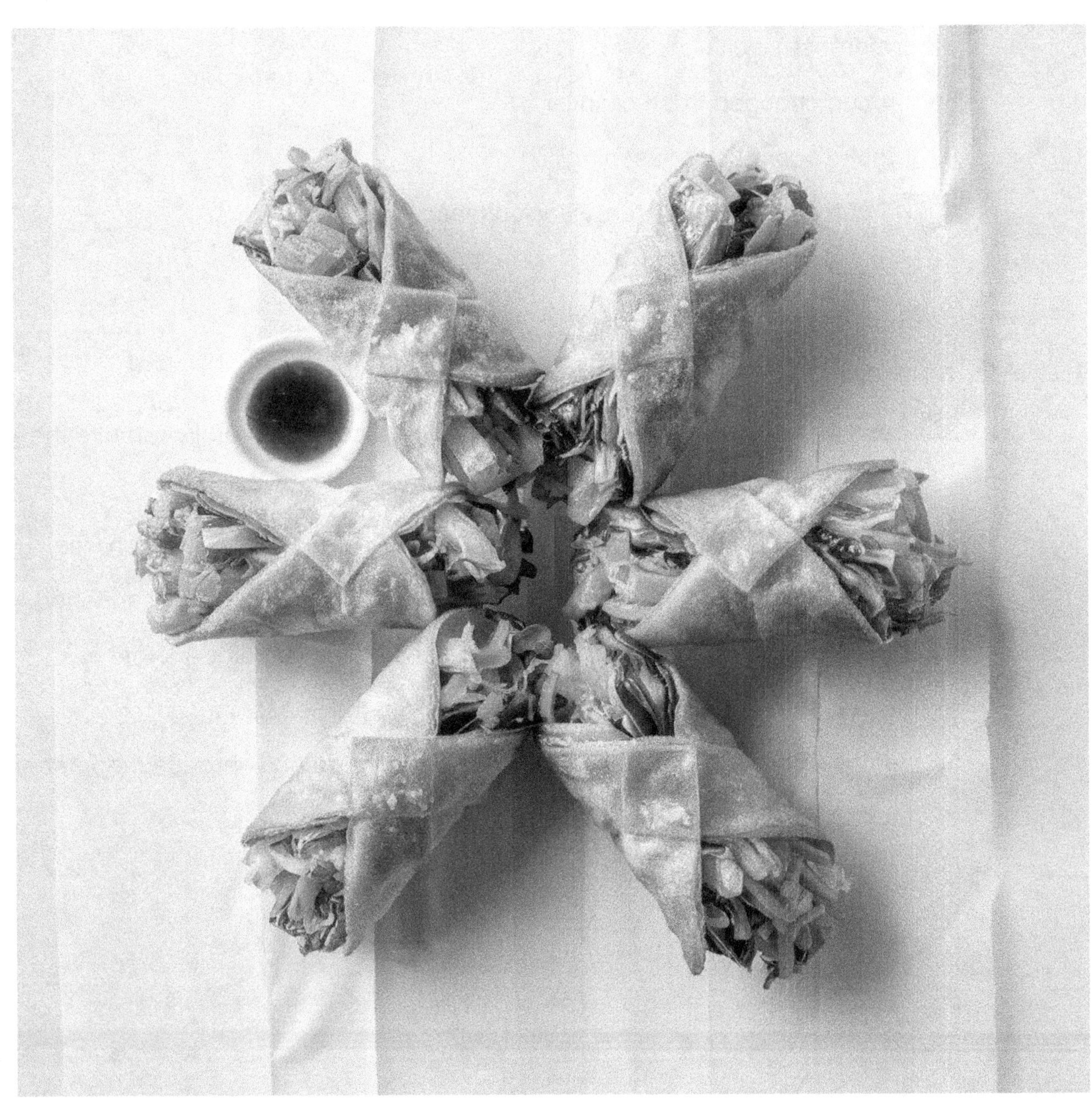

Ingredients:

- **For the Filling:**
    - 2 carrots, peeled and julienned (matchstick-thin slices)
    - 1/2 red bell pepper, deseeded and julienned
    - 1 green onion, thinly sliced (white and green parts)
    - 1 cup mung bean sprouts, rinsed and drained (optional)
    - 1/2 cup chopped cabbage (optional)
    - 1 clove garlic, minced
    - 2 tablespoons soy sauce (light or tamari for a gluten-free option)
    - 1 tablespoon rice vinegar
    - 1 tablespoon sesame oil
    - 1 teaspoon cornstarch mixed with 2 tablespoons water (cornstarch slurry)
    - Salt and freshly ground black pepper to taste
- **For the Wrappers:**
    - 1 package (20-24) round rice paper wrappers
    - Bowl of warm water (for dipping)
- **For Serving (Optional):**
    - Sweet and sour sauce
    - Chili garlic sauce
    - Peanut sauce (make your own or store-bought)

Instructions:

1. **Prepare the Filling:**
    - In a large bowl, combine julienned carrots, red bell pepper, green onion, mung bean sprouts (if using), and chopped cabbage (if using).

- Heat a wok or large skillet over medium heat. Add a drizzle of oil and saute the garlic for about 30 seconds, until fragrant.
- Add the vegetable mixture to the pan and cook for 2-3 minutes, stirring constantly, until slightly softened but still crisp-tender.
- In a small bowl, whisk together the soy sauce, rice vinegar, sesame oil, and cornstarch slurry.
- Pour the sauce mixture into the pan with the vegetables and cook for another minute, or until the sauce thickens slightly.
- Remove from heat and season with salt and pepper to taste. Let the filling cool completely before assembling the spring rolls.

2. **Assemble the Spring Rolls:**

   - Fill a shallow dish or bowl with warm water.
   - Dip a rice paper wrapper quickly into the warm water, just enough to soften it (about 5 seconds). Lay the softened wrapper on a clean work surface.
   - Place a heaping tablespoon of the cooled vegetable filling towards the bottom corner of the wrapper, diagonally.
   - Fold the bottom corner of the wrapper over the filling. Fold in the sides of the wrapper tightly towards the center.
   - Continue rolling up tightly, forming a cigar-shaped spring roll. Moisten the very end of the wrapper with a little water to seal it closed.
   - Repeat with remaining wrappers and filling.

3. **Cooking (Optional):**

   - You can enjoy these spring rolls fresh or lightly pan-fry them for a crispier texture.
   - To pan-fry: Heat a thin layer of oil in a skillet over medium heat. Fry the spring rolls for 1-2 minutes per side, or until golden brown and crispy.

- **Air-frying option:** Preheat your air fryer to 400°F (200°C). Lightly spray the spring rolls with cooking oil and cook for 5-7 minutes, or until golden brown and crispy, shaking the basket occasionally.

4. **Serve:**
   - Enjoy your vegetable spring rolls warm or at room temperature.
   - Serve with your favorite dipping sauces like sweet and sour sauce, chili garlic sauce, or peanut sauce.

Tips:

- You can customize the vegetables in the filling based on your preferences. Other options include shredded zucchini, mushrooms, or chopped water chestnuts.
- If you don't have rice paper wrappers, you can use spring roll wrappers found in the Asian section of most grocery stores. They may require a slightly different rolling technique.
- Leftover spring rolls can be stored in an airtight container in the refrigerator for up to 2 days. Reheat them in a pan or air fryer until warmed through.

Enjoy these delicious and healthy vegetable spring rolls!

Baked veggie samosas

Here's a recipe for delicious Baked Veggie Samosas, perfect for a PCOS-friendly snack or appetizer:

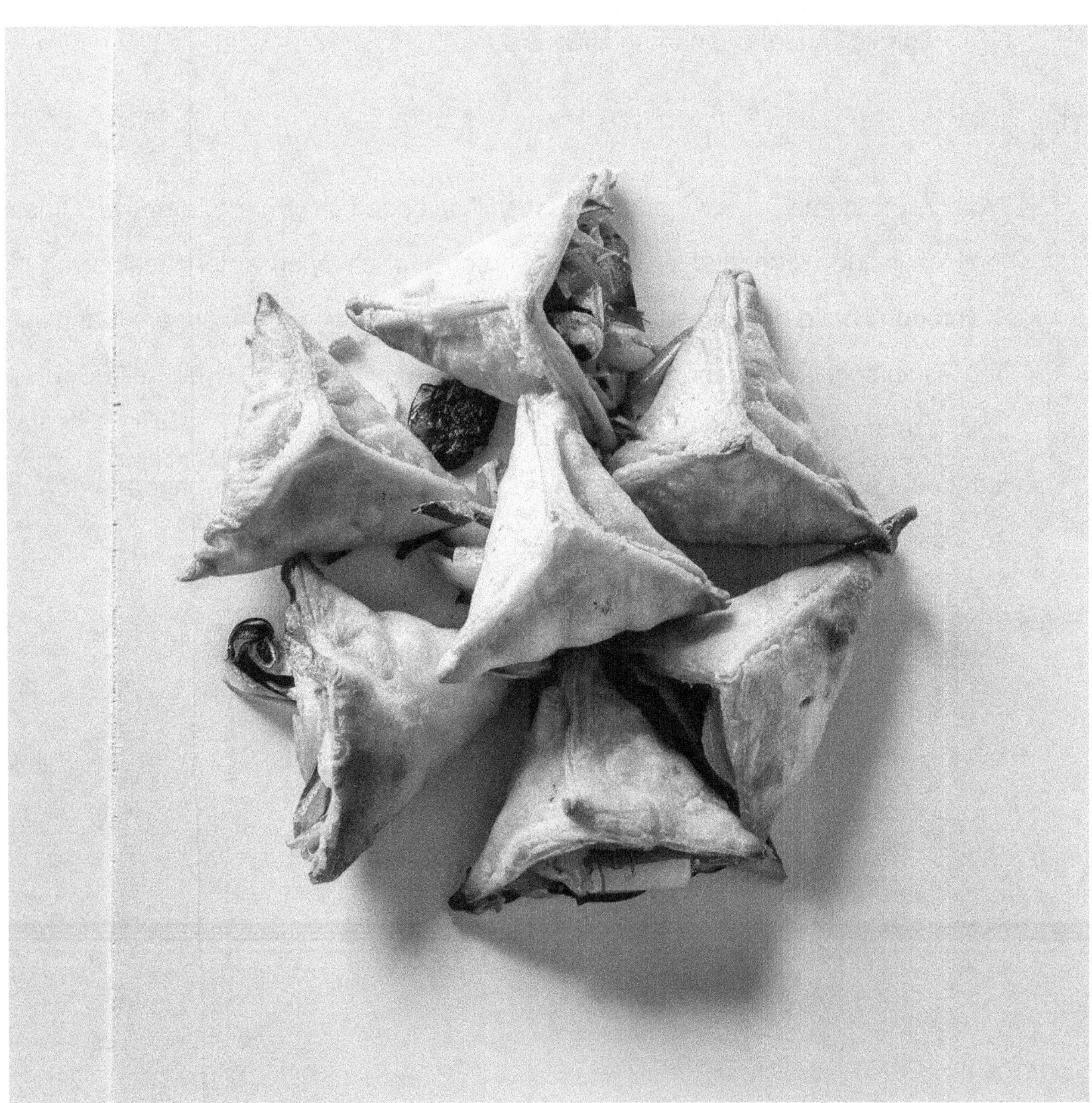

Ingredients:

- **For the Dough:**
    - 1 1/2 cups all-purpose flour (or gluten-free alternative)
    - 1/2 teaspoon baking powder
    - 1/2 teaspoon salt
    - 1/3 cup vegetable oil
    - 1/2 cup warm water (approximately)
- **For the Filling:**
    - 2 medium potatoes, peeled and diced
    - 1/2 cup frozen peas
    - 1/2 cup chopped carrots
    - 1/4 cup chopped onion
    - 1 tablespoon vegetable oil
    - 1 teaspoon cumin seeds
    - 1/2 teaspoon coriander powder
    - 1/4 teaspoon turmeric powder
    - 1/4 teaspoon chili powder (adjust to your spice preference)
    - 1/4 teaspoon garam masala (optional)
    - Salt and freshly ground black pepper to taste
    - 1 tablespoon chopped fresh cilantro (optional)
- **For Baking:**
    - Cooking spray
    - Sesame seeds (optional, for garnish)

Instructions:

1. **Make the Dough:**

- In a large bowl, whisk together the flour, baking powder, and salt.
- Add the vegetable oil and mix it in using your fingertips until crumbly.
- Gradually add the warm water, a tablespoon at a time, mixing until a soft dough forms. You may not need all the water.
- Knead the dough on a lightly floured surface for 5 minutes, or until smooth and elastic.
- Cover the dough with a damp cloth and let it rest for 30 minutes at room temperature.

2. **Prepare the Filling:**

- In a large pot, boil the diced potatoes until tender, about 10-12 minutes. Drain and set aside.
- While the potatoes are cooking, heat the vegetable oil in a skillet over medium heat.
- Add the cumin seeds and cook for 30 seconds, until fragrant.
- Add the chopped onion and carrots to the pan and cook for 5 minutes, or until softened.
- Stir in the turmeric powder, coriander powder, chili powder, and garam masala (if using). Cook for another minute, allowing the spices to bloom.
- Add the cooked and drained potatoes, frozen peas, and salt and pepper to taste. Stir to combine and heat through for another 2-3 minutes.
- Remove from heat and stir in the chopped cilantro (if using). Let the filling cool slightly before assembling the samosas.

3. **Assemble and Bake:**

- Preheat the oven to 400°F (200°C). Line a baking sheet with parchment paper.
- Divide the dough into 12 equal balls. Roll out each ball on a lightly floured surface into a thin circle, about 5-6 inches in diameter.

- Place a heaping tablespoon of the cooled filling in the center of each dough circle.
- Moisten the edges of the dough circle with a little water. Fold one half of the circle over the filling to form a semi-circle. Press the edges together to seal the samosa. You can crimp the edges with a fork for a decorative touch.
- Place the assembled samosas on the prepared baking sheet, leaving some space between them.
- Lightly spray the tops of the samosas with cooking spray. Sprinkle with sesame seeds (optional) for garnish.

4. **Bake:**

- Bake the samosas for 20-25 minutes, or until golden brown and crispy.
- Let the samosas cool slightly before serving.

5. **Serve:**

- Enjoy your baked veggie samosas warm with your favorite dipping sauce like chutney or yogurt dip.

Tips:

- You can adjust the vegetables in the filling based on your preferences. Other options include chopped bell peppers, green beans, or corn.
- If the dough becomes too sticky while rolling, add a little more flour, one tablespoon at a time, until manageable.
- Leftover baked samosas can be stored in an airtight container in the refrigerator for up to 3 days. Reheat them in a preheated oven or air fryer until warmed through and crispy again.

These baked veggie samosas are a delicious and healthy alternative to traditional fried samosas. Enjoy!

Mini quiches

Mini quiches are delightful bite-sized treats perfect for PCOS-friendly snacks, appetizers, or even light meals. They're easily customizable and can be enjoyed warm or at room temperature. Here are two recipe ideas to inspire your mini quiche creations:

Classic Ham and Cheese Mini Quiches:

This recipe offers a familiar and satisfying flavor combination.

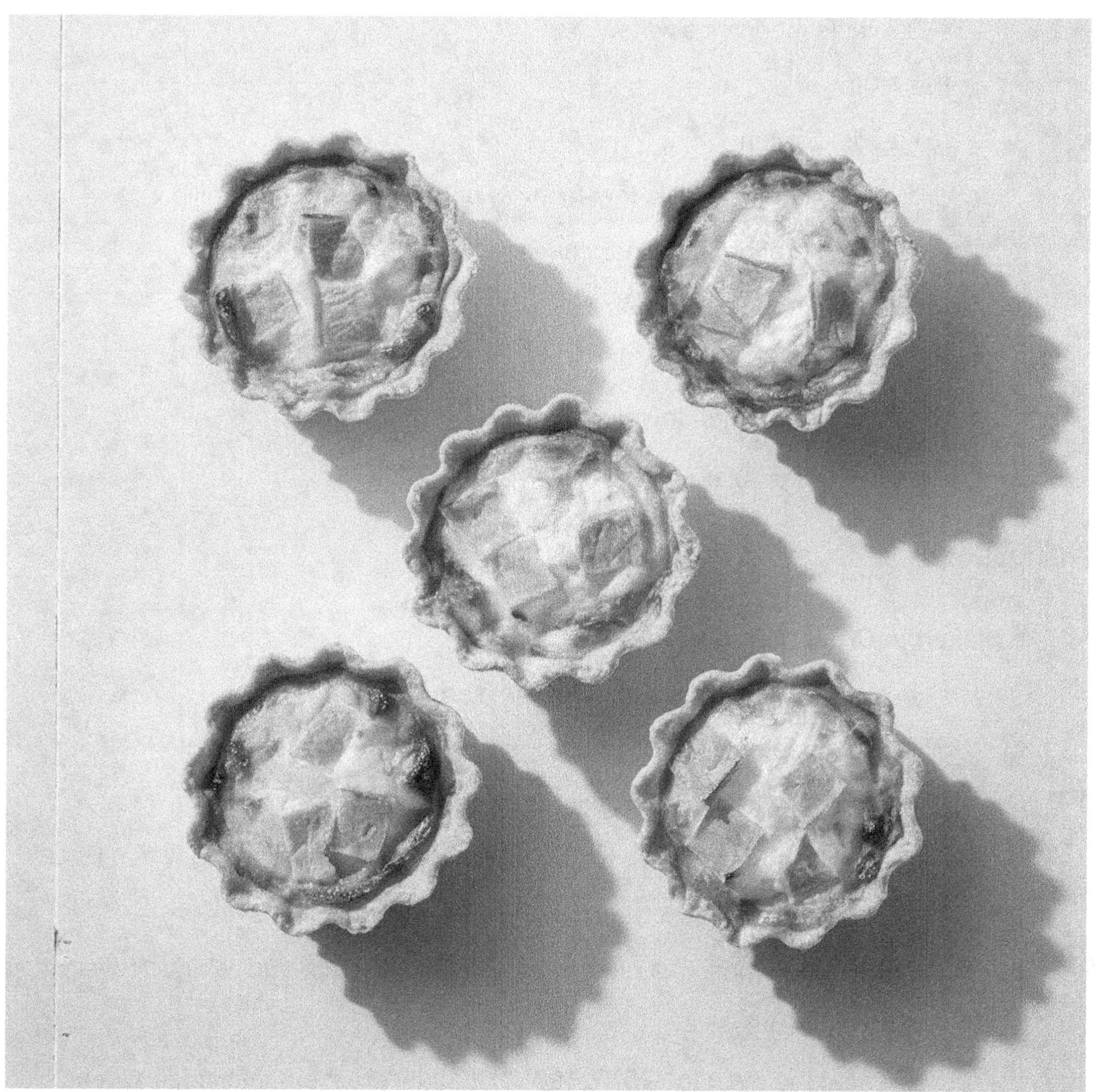

Ingredients:

- **For the Crust (Makes about 24 mini quiche shells):**
    - 1 1/2 cups all-purpose flour (or gluten-free alternative for a crustless option)
    - 1/2 teaspoon salt
    - 1/2 cup cold unsalted butter, cubed

- o   3-4 tablespoons ice water
- **For the Filling:**
  - o   4 eggs, beaten
  - o   1 cup milk (whole milk, low-fat milk, or unsweetened nut milk)
  - o   1/2 cup shredded cheddar cheese
  - o   1/4 cup diced cooked ham
  - o   1/4 cup chopped onion
  - o   1/4 teaspoon dried thyme
  - o   Salt and freshly ground black pepper to taste

Instructions:

1. **Make the Crust (Optional):**
   - o   In a large bowl, whisk together the flour and salt.
   - o   Using a pastry cutter or your fingertips, cut the cold butter into the flour mixture until it resembles coarse crumbs.
   - o   Gradually add the ice water, a tablespoon at a time, tossing with a fork until the dough just comes together. Be careful not to overmix.
   - o   Form the dough into a disc, wrap it in plastic wrap, and refrigerate for at least 30 minutes.
   - o   Preheat the oven to 375°F (190°C). Lightly grease a mini muffin pan.
2. **Assemble the Mini Quiches:**
   - o   On a lightly floured surface, roll out the chilled dough to a thickness of about 1/8 inch.
   - o   Using a round cookie cutter or a glass, cut out circles of dough slightly larger than the diameter of your mini muffin cups.
   - o   Gently press the dough circles into the greased muffin cups, forming little tart shells.

- If you're not using a crust, simply grease the mini muffin cups.

3. **Prepare the Filling:**

   - In a large bowl, whisk together the beaten eggs and milk.
   - Stir in the shredded cheddar cheese, diced cooked ham, chopped onion, and dried thyme.
   - Season with salt and pepper to taste.

4. **Bake:**

   - Pour the egg mixture evenly into the prepared mini quiche shells or greased muffin cups.
   - Bake for 20-25 minutes, or until the egg filling is set and the crust is golden brown (if using).

5. **Serve:**

   - Let the mini quiches cool slightly before serving.
   - Enjoy them warm or at room temperature.

Spinach and Feta Mini Quiches (Vegetarian Option):

This recipe provides a vegetarian twist with a burst of spinach and creamy feta.

Ingredients:

- **For the Crust (Optional, follow instructions above):**
  - Same ingredients and instructions as the Classic Ham and Cheese Mini Quiches.
- **For the Filling:**
  - 4 eggs, beaten
  - 1 cup milk (whole milk, low-fat milk, or unsweetened nut milk)
  - 1/2 cup crumbled feta cheese
  - 1/2 cup chopped fresh spinach

- 1/4 cup chopped red onion
- 1/4 teaspoon dried nutmeg
- Salt and freshly ground black pepper to taste

Instructions:

1. Follow steps 1-3 from the Classic Ham and Cheese Mini Quiches recipe to prepare the crust (optional) and assemble the mini quiches.
2. **Prepare the Filling:**
   - In a large bowl, whisk together the beaten eggs and milk.
   - Stir in the crumbled feta cheese, chopped fresh spinach, chopped red onion, and dried nutmeg.
   - Season with salt and pepper to taste.
3. **Bake:**
   - Follow step 4 from the Classic Ham and Cheese Mini Quiches recipe to bake the mini quiches.
4. **Serve:**
   - Follow step 5 from the Classic Ham and Cheese Mini Quiches recipe to serve.

Tips:

- You can customize the fillings with your favorite ingredients. Some ideas include chopped broccoli and cheddar cheese, crumbled sausage and peppers, or mushrooms and Swiss cheese.
- Pre-bake the crusts for 10 minutes at 375°F (190°C) before adding the filling if you're using a thicker dough to prevent soggy bottoms.

Chicken skewers with a healthy marinade

Lemon Herb Chicken Skewers

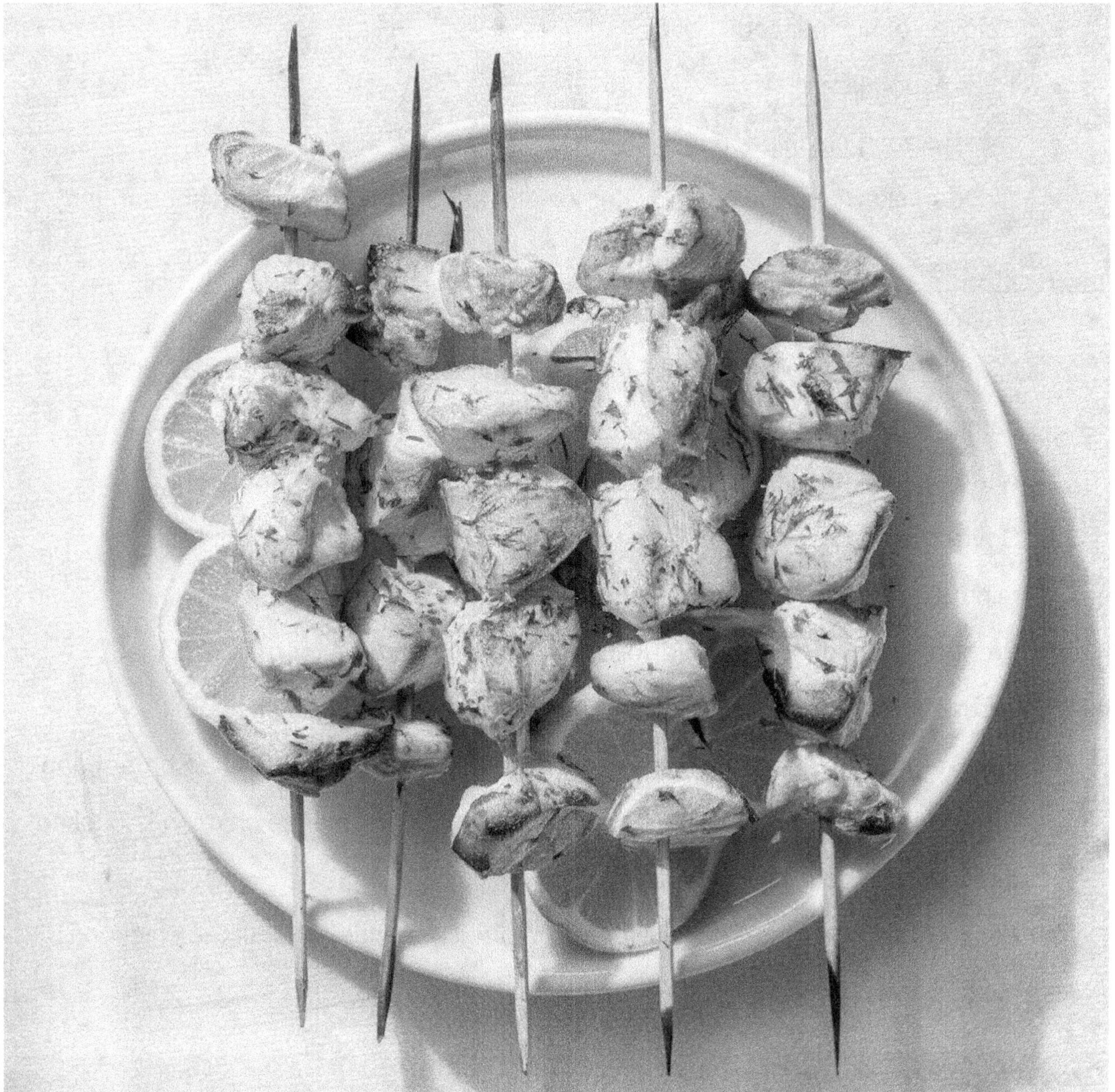

Ingredients:

- 1 pound boneless, skinless chicken breasts or thighs, cut into bite-sized pieces
- 1/4 cup fresh lemon juice

* 2 tablespoons olive oil
* 1 tablespoon chopped fresh thyme
* 1 tablespoon chopped fresh rosemary
* 1 tablespoon chopped fresh parsley
* 2 cloves garlic, minced
* 1/2 teaspoon salt
* 1/4 teaspoon black pepper
* Wooden skewers (soaked in water for at least 30 minutes to prevent burning)

Instructions:

1. In a large bowl, whisk together the lemon juice, olive oil, thyme, rosemary, parsley, garlic, salt, and pepper.
2. Add the chicken pieces to the marinade and toss to coat them evenly.
3. Cover the bowl and marinate the chicken in the refrigerator for at least 30 minutes, or up to 4 hours for deeper flavor.
4. Preheat the oven to 400°F (200°C) or prepare your grill for medium heat.
5. Thread the marinated chicken pieces onto soaked wooden skewers.
6. **For Baking:** Arrange the skewers on a baking sheet lined with parchment paper. Bake for 15-20 minutes, flipping halfway through, or until the chicken is cooked through and the juices run clear.
7. **For Grilling:** Grill the skewers for 5-7 minutes per side, or until the chicken is cooked through and the juices run clear.

Greek Yogurt Marinade Chicken Skewers:

This recipe uses Greek yogurt for a protein-rich and flavorful marinade.

Ingredients:

- 1 pound boneless, skinless chicken breasts or thighs, cut into bite-sized pieces
- 1 cup plain Greek yogurt (2% or higher fat content)
- 1/4 cup lemon juice
- 2 tablespoons olive oil
- 1 tablespoon chopped fresh oregano
- 1 tablespoon chopped fresh mint
- 1 teaspoon dried thyme
- 1/2 teaspoon garlic powder
- 1/2 teaspoon salt
- 1/4 teaspoon black pepper
- Wooden skewers (soaked in water for at least 30 minutes to prevent burning)

Instructions:

1. In a large bowl, whisk together the Greek yogurt, lemon juice, olive oil, oregano, mint, thyme, garlic powder, salt, and pepper.
2. Add the chicken pieces to the marinade and toss to coat them evenly.
3. Cover the bowl and marinate the chicken in the refrigerator for at least 30 minutes, or up to 4 hours for deeper flavor.
4. Preheat the oven to 400°F (200°C) or prepare your grill for medium heat.
5. Thread the marinated chicken pieces onto soaked wooden skewers.
6. **For Baking:** Arrange the skewers on a baking sheet lined with parchment paper. Bake for 15-20 minutes, flipping halfway through, or until the chicken is cooked through and the juices run clear.
7. **For Grilling:** Grill the skewers for 5-7 minutes per side, or until the chicken is cooked through and the juices run clear.

Tips:

- You can use chicken thighs for a juicier result, but adjust the cooking time accordingly as they may take a few minutes longer to cook through.
- Feel free to experiment with different herbs and spices in the marinades to create your own flavor variations.
- Serve the chicken skewers with your favorite dipping sauce, such as tzatziki sauce, chimichurri sauce, or a simple lemon-herb yogurt sauce.
- Leftover chicken skewers can be stored in an airtight container in the refrigerator for up to 3 days. Reheat them in the oven or microwave until warmed through.

Enjoy these delicious and healthy chicken skewers with a healthy marinade!

Shrimp cocktail with a low-fat avocado crema

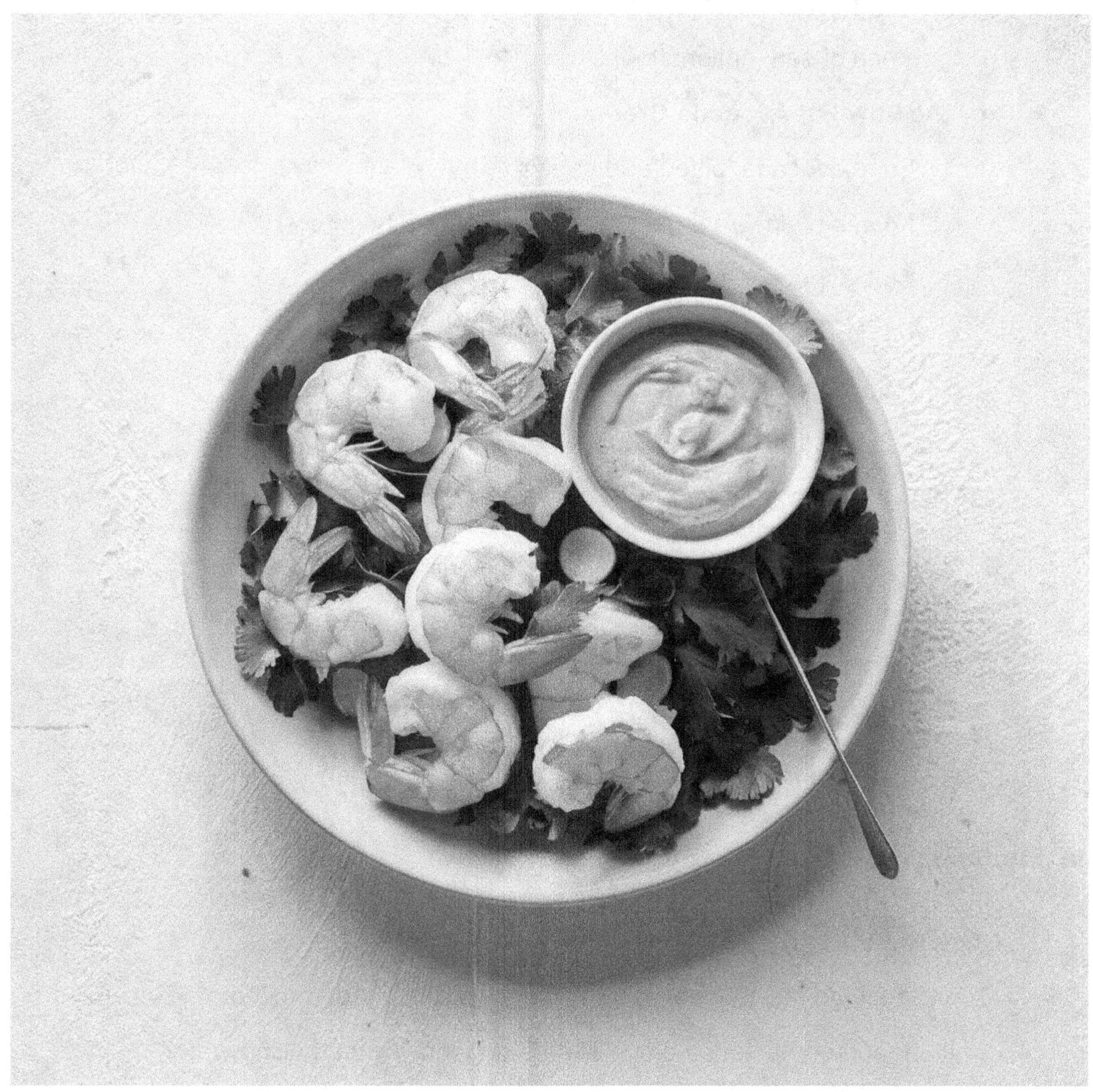

Ingredients:

- **For the Shrimp:**
    - 1 pound large shrimp, peeled and deveined
    - Water
    - 1 tablespoon lemon juice

- o 1/2 teaspoon dried dill

- o 1/4 teaspoon black peppercorns

- o Pinch of salt (optional)

- **For the Low-Fat Avocado Crema:**

  - o 1 ripe avocado, pitted and peeled

  - o 1/4 cup plain Greek yogurt (2% or higher fat content)

  - o 1 tablespoon lemon juice

  - o 1/4 cup chopped fresh cilantro

  - o 1 clove garlic, minced

  - o Salt and freshly ground black pepper to taste

- **For Serving:**

  - o Cocktail glasses or bowls

  - o Ice (optional)

  - o Lemon wedges for garnish

  - o Cocktail sauce (optional)

  - o Chopped fresh herbs like parsley or dill (optional)

Instructions:

1. **Cook the Shrimp:**

   - o In a medium saucepan, bring water to a boil. Add the lemon juice, dill, peppercorns, and a pinch of salt (optional) to the boiling water.

   - o Reduce heat to medium-low and simmer for 5 minutes to infuse the flavor into the water.

   - o Add the shrimp and cook for 2-3 minutes, or until the shrimp turn pink and opaque. Do not overcook, or they will become rubbery.

   - o Drain the shrimp and rinse them under cold water to stop the cooking process. Set aside to cool completely.

2. **Make the Low-Fat Avocado Crema:**

    - In a blender or food processor, combine the avocado, Greek yogurt, lemon juice, chopped cilantro, and minced garlic.
    - Blend until smooth and creamy. Season with salt and pepper to taste.

3. **Assemble and Serve:**

    - Fill cocktail glasses or bowls with ice (optional).
    - Arrange the cooked and cooled shrimp in the glasses.
    - Pour the avocado crema over the shrimp, leaving some room at the top.
    - Garnish with lemon wedges, chopped fresh herbs (optional), and a drizzle of cocktail sauce (optional).

Tips:

- You can poach the shrimp instead of boiling them for a more delicate flavor.
- For a spicier crema, add a pinch of red pepper flakes or a chopped jalapeno pepper to the blender with the other crema ingredients.
- Pre-cooked frozen shrimp can be used for convenience. Thaw them completely before using.
- Leftover avocado crema can be stored in an airtight container in the refrigerator for up to 1 day. However, the color may brown slightly due to avocado oxidation.

Enjoy this refreshing and healthy shrimp cocktail with a delicious low-fat avocado crema!

Vegetarian and Veggies

Vegetable Spring Rolls

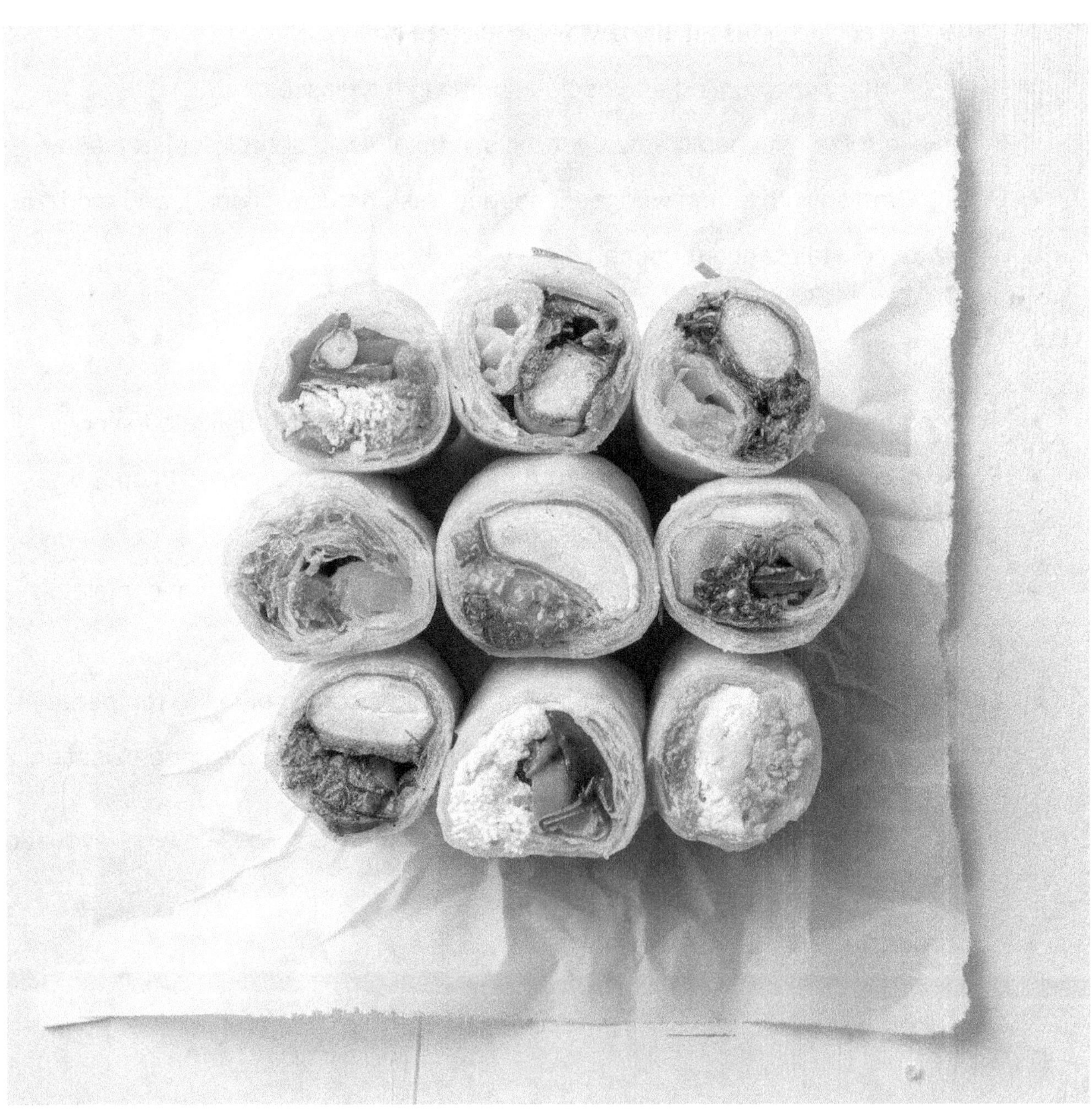

Servings: Makes about 20-24 spring rolls (depending on size)

Preparation Time: 20 minutes

Cooking Time: (Optional) 2-4 minutes per side for pan-frying or 5-7 minutes per side for air-frying

Ingredients:

- **For the Filling:**
    - 2 carrots, julienned (matchstick-thin slices)
    - 1/2 red bell pepper, deseeded and julienned
    - 1 green onion, thinly sliced (white and green parts)
    - 1 cup mung bean sprouts, rinsed and drained (optional)
    - 1/2 cup chopped cabbage (optional)
    - 1 clove garlic, minced
    - 2 tablespoons soy sauce (light or tamari for a gluten-free option)
    - 1 tablespoon rice vinegar
    - 1 tablespoon sesame oil
    - 1 teaspoon cornstarch mixed with 2 tablespoons water (cornstarch slurry)
    - Salt and freshly ground black pepper to taste
- **For the Wrappers:**
    - 1 package (20-24) round rice paper wrappers
    - Bowl of warm water (for dipping)
- **For Serving (Optional):**
    - Sweet and sour sauce
    - Chili garlic sauce
    - Peanut sauce (make your own or store-bought)

Instructions:

1. **Prepare the Filling (10 minutes):**
   - In a large bowl, combine julienned carrots, red bell pepper, green onion, mung bean sprouts (if using), and chopped cabbage (if using).
   - Heat a wok or large skillet over medium heat. Add a drizzle of oil and saute the garlic for about 30 seconds, until fragrant.
   - Add the vegetable mixture to the pan and cook for 2-3 minutes, stirring constantly, until slightly softened but still crisp-tender.
   - In a small bowl, whisk together the soy sauce, rice vinegar, sesame oil, and cornstarch slurry.
   - Pour the sauce mixture into the pan with the vegetables and cook for another minute, or until the sauce thickens slightly.
   - Remove from heat and season with salt and pepper to taste. Let the filling cool completely before assembling the spring rolls.
2. **Assemble the Spring Rolls (5-10 minutes):**
   - Fill a shallow dish or bowl with warm water.
   - Dip a rice paper wrapper quickly into the warm water, just enough to soften it (about 5 seconds). Lay the softened wrapper on a clean work surface.
   - Place a heaping tablespoon of the cooled vegetable filling towards the bottom corner of the wrapper, diagonally.
   - Fold the bottom corner of the wrapper over the filling. Fold in the sides of the wrapper tightly towards the center.
   - Continue rolling up tightly, forming a cigar-shaped spring roll. Moisten the very end of the wrapper with a little water to seal it closed.
   - Repeat with remaining wrappers and filling.

3. **Cooking (Optional, 2-4 minutes per side for pan-frying or 5-7 minutes per side for air-frying):**
   - You can enjoy these spring rolls fresh or lightly pan-fry them for a crispier texture.
   - To pan-fry: Heat a thin layer of oil in a skillet over medium heat. Fry the spring rolls for 1-2 minutes per side, or until golden brown and crispy.
   - Air-frying option: Preheat your air fryer to 400°F (200°C). Lightly spray the spring rolls with cooking oil and cook for 5-7 minutes, or until golden brown and crispy, shaking the basket occasionally.
4. **Serve (enjoy immediately):**
   - Enjoy your vegetable spring rolls warm or at room temperature.
   - Serve with your favorite dipping sauces like sweet and sour sauce, chili garlic sauce, or peanut sauce.

Tips:

- You can customize the vegetables in the filling based on your preferences. Other options include shredded zucchini, mushrooms, or chopped water chestnuts.
- If you don't have rice paper wrappers, you can use spring roll wrappers found in the Asian section of most grocery stores. They may require a slightly different rolling technique.
- Leftover spring rolls can be stored in an airtight container in the refrigerator for up to 2 days. Reheat them in a pan or air fryer until warmed through.

Enjoy these delicious and healthy vegetable spring rolls!

Stuffed Mini Peppers

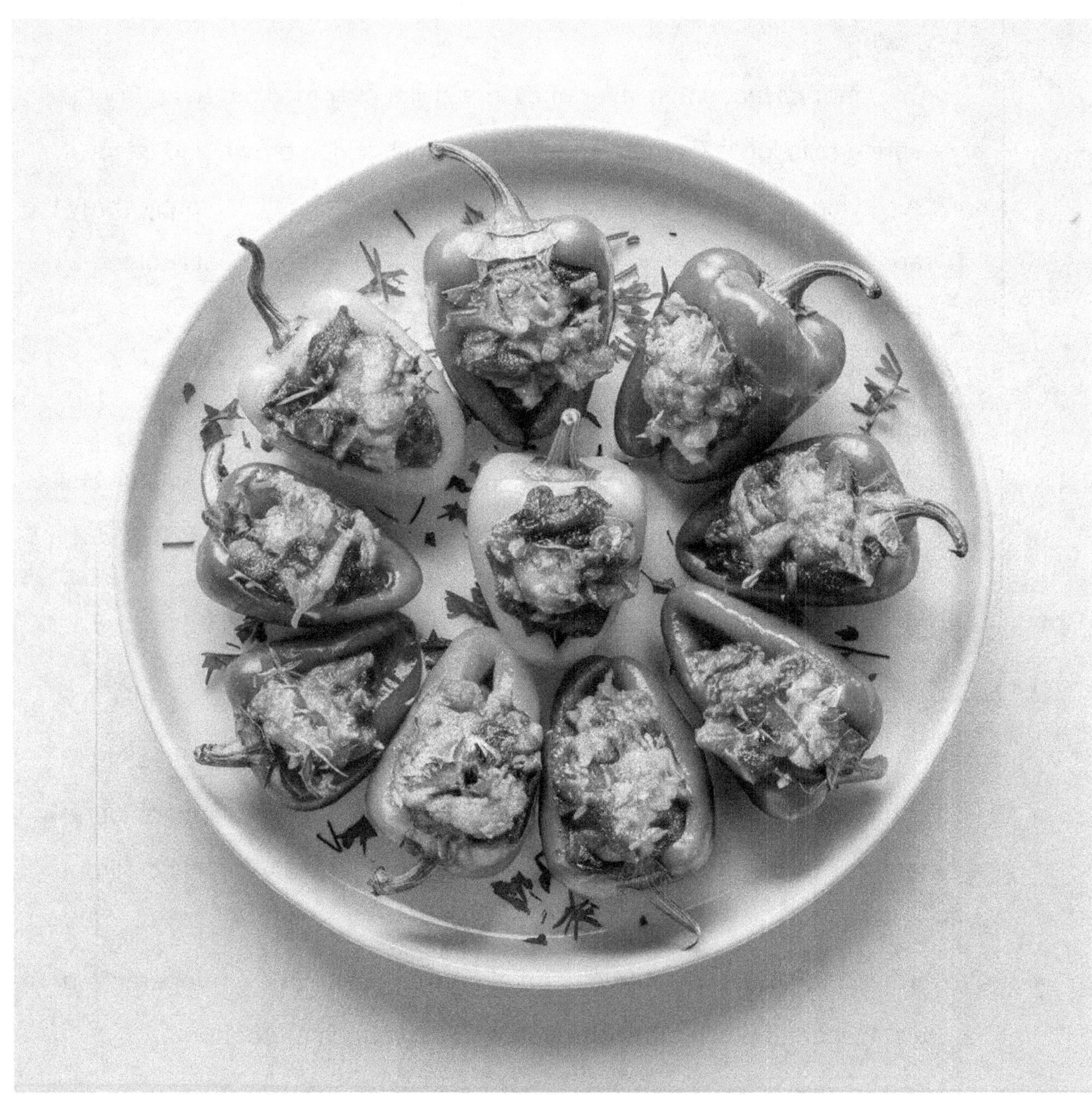

Ingredients:

- **For the Filling (enough for 12-15 mini peppers):**
    - 1 tablespoon olive oil
    - 1/2 onion, chopped
    - 1 clove garlic, minced
    - 1 cup chopped mushrooms (optional)
    - 1 cup cooked quinoa (or brown rice)
    - 1/2 cup black beans, rinsed and drained
    - 1/2 cup chopped corn (fresh or frozen)
    - 1/4 cup chopped fresh cilantro
    - 1/4 cup chopped fresh parsley
    - 1 tablespoon tomato paste
    - 1 teaspoon ground cumin
    - 1/2 teaspoon chili powder (adjust to your spice preference)
    - Salt and freshly ground black pepper to taste
    - 1/2 cup shredded cheddar cheese (optional)
- **For the Mini Peppers:**
    - 12-15 mini bell peppers (assorted colors for visual appeal, optional)
    - Olive oil spray

Instructions:

Preparation Time: 15 minutes **Cooking Time:** 20-25 minutes

1. **Prepare the Filling (15 minutes):**
    - Heat olive oil in a large skillet over medium heat. Add the chopped onion and cook for 3-4 minutes, or until softened.
    - Add the minced garlic and cook for another minute, until fragrant.

- If using mushrooms, add them to the pan and cook for an additional 5 minutes, or until softened and slightly browned.
  - Stir in the cooked quinoa (or brown rice), black beans, chopped corn, chopped cilantro, and chopped parsley.
  - Add the tomato paste, ground cumin, chili powder, salt, and pepper to taste. Mix well and cook for 2-3 minutes, or until heated through.
  - If using shredded cheese, stir it into the filling and cook until melted (optional).

2. **Prepare the Mini Peppers (5 minutes):**
   - Preheat the oven to 400°F (200°C). Lightly grease a baking sheet with olive oil spray.
   - Wash the mini peppers and cut them in half lengthwise, removing the seeds and membranes.

3. **Assemble and Bake (20-25 minutes):**
   - Spoon the filling evenly into the prepared mini pepper halves.
   - Arrange the filled peppers on the greased baking sheet.
   - Bake for 20-25 minutes, or until the peppers are tender and the filling is heated through.

4. **Serve (enjoy immediately):**
   - Let the stuffed mini peppers cool slightly before serving.
   - Enjoy them warm as an appetizer, light meal, or side dish.

Tips:

- You can customize the vegetables in the filling based on your preferences. Other options include chopped zucchini, chopped bell peppers of a different color, or diced tomatoes.

- If you don't have cooked quinoa or brown rice, you can use another cooked grain like chopped barley or chopped farro.
- Leftover stuffed mini peppers can be stored in an airtight container in the refrigerator for up to 3 days. Reheat them in a preheated oven or microwave until warmed through.

These stuffed mini peppers are a delicious and healthy way to incorporate more vegetables into your vegetarian and veggie diet!

Mini Quiches

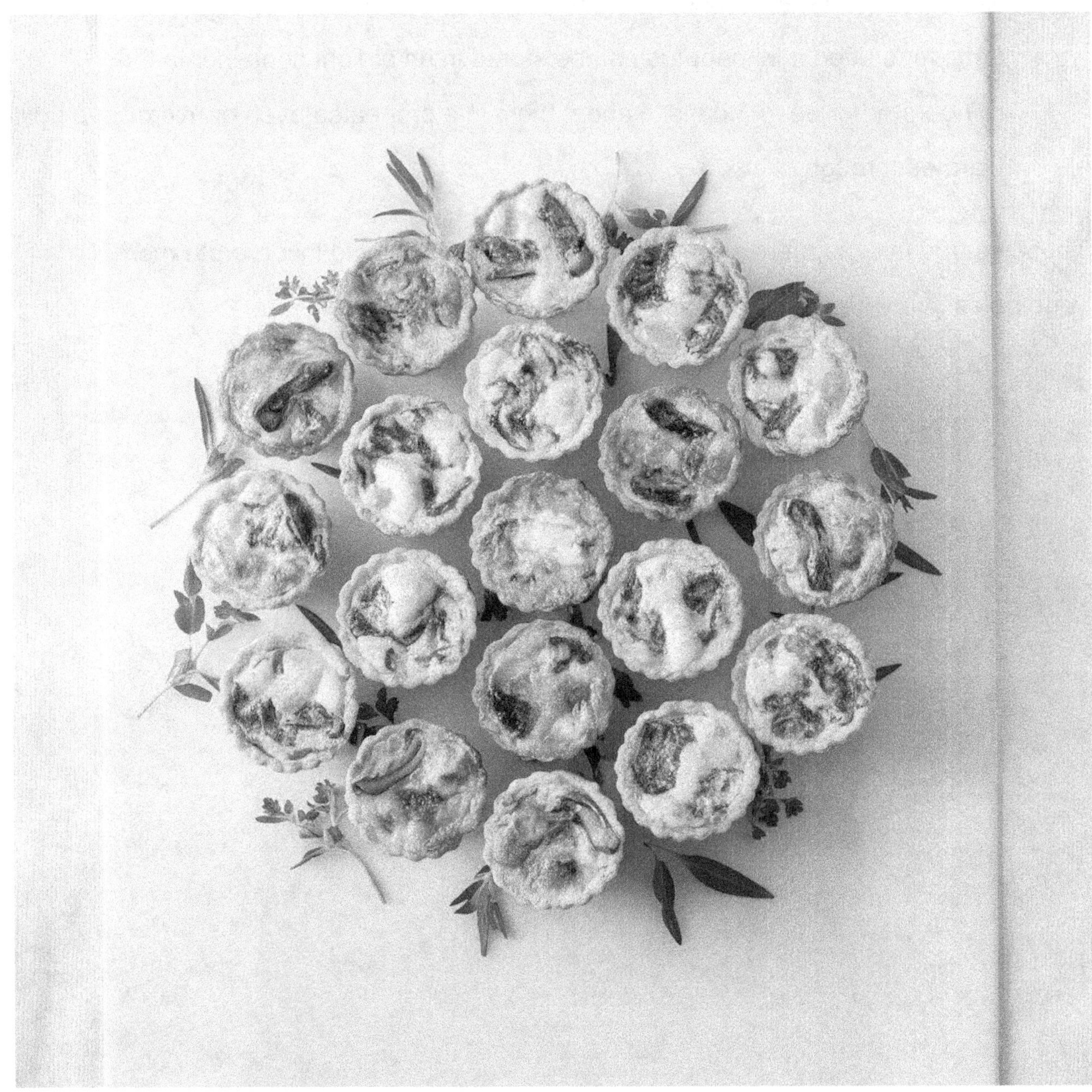

Mini quiches are delightful bite-sized treats perfect for vegetarian and veggie meals, appetizers, or even light snacks. They're easily customizable with a variety of fillings, and this recipe provides two delicious options:

Crustless Mini Quiches (Makes about 12)

Preparation Time: 15 minutes **Cooking Time:** 20-25 minutes

Ingredients:

- **For the Filling:**
    - 4 eggs, beaten
    - 1 cup milk (whole milk, low-fat milk, or unsweetened nut milk)
    - 1 cup shredded cheddar cheese (or your favorite cheese)
    - 1/2 cup chopped vegetables (such as broccoli, spinach, mushrooms, or bell peppers)
    - 1/4 cup chopped onion
    - 1/4 teaspoon dried thyme (or other herbs like oregano or basil)
    - Salt and freshly ground black pepper to taste

Instructions:

1. **Preheat the oven to 375°F (190°C).** Grease a 12-cup muffin tin.
2. **Prepare the Filling (10 minutes):**
    - In a large bowl, whisk together the beaten eggs and milk.
    - Stir in the shredded cheese, chopped vegetables, chopped onion, dried thyme, salt, and pepper.
3. **Assemble and Bake (10-15 minutes prep, 20-25 minutes baking):**
    - Pour the egg mixture evenly into the greased muffin cups.
    - Bake for 20-25 minutes, or until the egg filling is set and the tops are golden brown.
4. **Serve (enjoy warm or at room temperature):**
    - Let the mini quiches cool slightly in the muffin tin before serving.
    - Enjoy them warm or at room temperature.

Tips:

- Get creative with your fillings! You can use a variety of chopped vegetables, cooked lentils or black beans, or crumbled tofu for a protein boost.
- If you prefer a richer flavor, add a tablespoon of grated Parmesan cheese to the filling.
- Leftover mini quiches can be stored in an airtight container in the refrigerator for up to 3 days. Reheat them in the oven or microwave until warmed through.

Mini Quiches with a Buttery Crust (Makes about 12)

Preparation Time: 30 minutes (including chilling time for dough) **Cooking Time:** 10-15 minutes (pre-bake) + 15-20 minutes (bake with filling)

Ingredients:

- **For the Crust:**
    - 1 1/2 cups all-purpose flour
    - 1/2 teaspoon salt
    - 1/2 cup cold unsalted butter, cubed
    - 3-4 tablespoons ice water
- **For the Filling:**
    - Same ingredients and instructions as the Crustless Mini Quiches recipe above.

Instructions:

1. **Make the Crust (20 minutes):**
    - In a large bowl, whisk together the flour and salt.

- Using a pastry cutter or your fingertips, cut the cold butter into the flour mixture until it resembles coarse crumbs.
- Gradually add the ice water, a tablespoon at a time, tossing with a fork until the dough just comes together. Be careful not to overmix.
- Form the dough into a disc, wrap it in plastic wrap, and refrigerate for at least 30 minutes.

2. **Preheat the oven to 375°F (190°C).** Lightly grease a 12-cup muffin tin.

3. **Prepare the Filling (10 minutes):**
   - Follow steps 2 and 3 from the Crustless Mini Quiches recipe above to prepare the filling.

4. **Assemble and Bake (10-15 minutes prep, 25-35 minutes baking):**
   - On a lightly floured surface, roll out the chilled dough to a thickness of about 1/8 inch.
   - Using a round cookie cutter or a glass, cut out circles of dough slightly larger than the diameter of your muffin cups.
   - Gently press the dough circles into the greased muffin cups, forming little tart shells.

Lentil Soup

Here's a delicious lentil soup recipe packed with protein and fiber, perfect for a vegetarian diet:

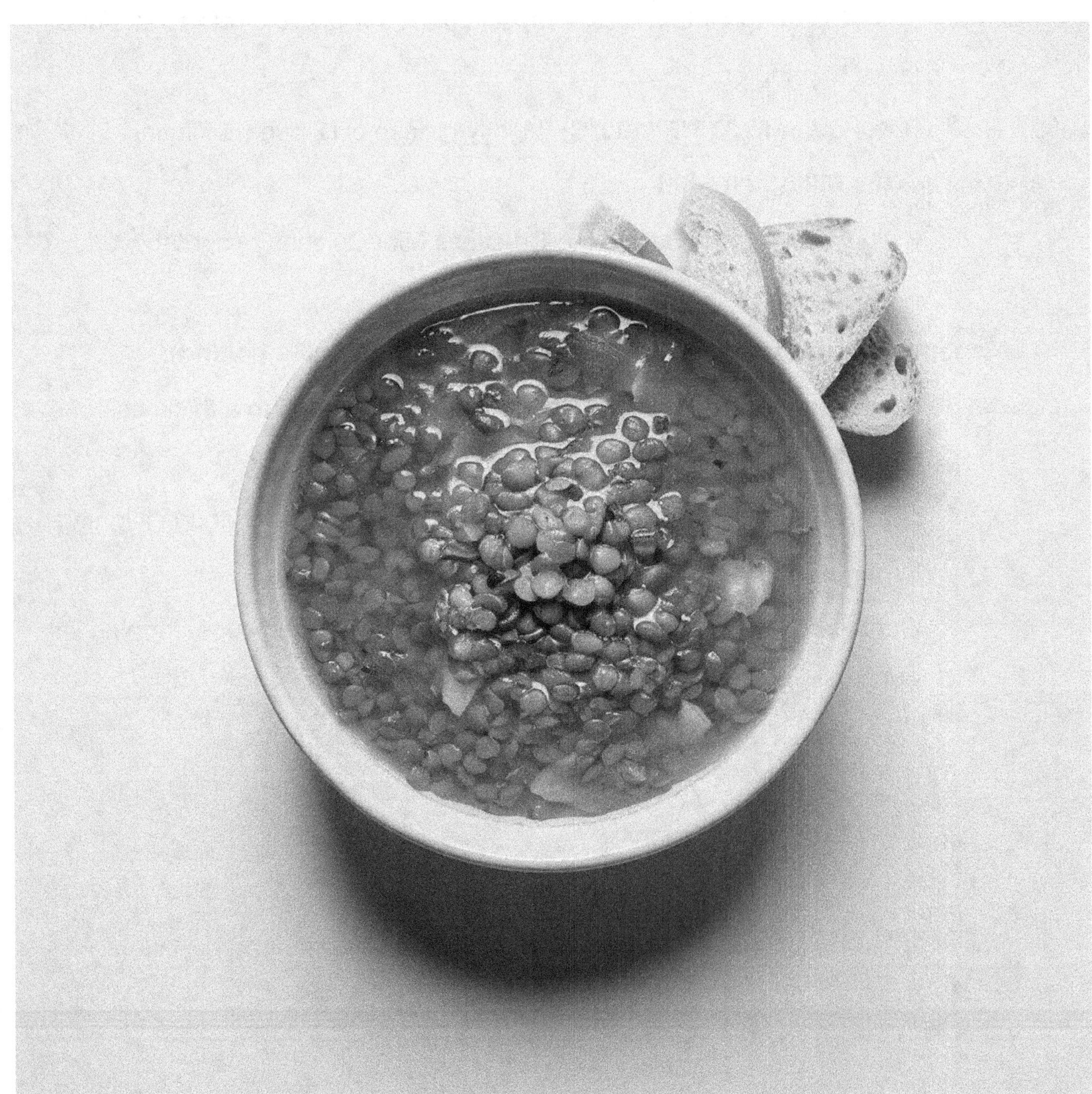

Ingredients:

- **For the Soup:**
  - 1 tablespoon olive oil
  - 1 onion, chopped
  - 2 carrots, chopped (about 1 cup)
  - 2 celery stalks, chopped (about 1 cup)
  - 2 cloves garlic, minced
  - 1 teaspoon ground cumin
  - 1/2 teaspoon dried thyme
  - 1/4 teaspoon red pepper flakes (optional, adjust for spice preference)
  - 1 cup brown or green lentils, rinsed
  - 4 cups vegetable broth
  - 1 (14.5-ounce) can diced tomatoes, undrained
  - 1 cup chopped kale or spinach
  - 1 teaspoon salt, or to taste
  - Freshly ground black pepper to taste
- **For Serving (Optional):**
  - Lemon wedges
  - Chopped fresh parsley
  - Crusty bread

Instructions:

Preparation Time: 10 minutes **Cooking Time:** 30-35 minutes

1. **Sauté the Vegetables (5 minutes):**
   - Heat olive oil in a large pot or Dutch oven over medium heat.

o Add the chopped onion, carrots, and celery. Sauté for 5 minutes, or until softened.

2. **Add Spices and Aromatics (1 minute):**

   o Stir in the minced garlic, ground cumin, dried thyme, and red pepper flakes (if using). Cook for another minute, until fragrant.

3. **Simmer with Lentils and Broth (20-25 minutes):**

   o Add the rinsed lentils, vegetable broth, and diced tomatoes (with their juices) to the pot.

   o Bring to a boil, then reduce heat and simmer for 20-25 minutes, or until the lentils are tender but still hold their shape.

4. **Add Greens and Seasonings (5 minutes):**

   o Stir in the chopped kale or spinach and cook for 5 minutes, or until wilted.

   o Season with salt and freshly ground black pepper to taste.

5. **Serve (enjoy warm):**

   o Ladle the lentil soup into bowls and serve hot.

   o Garnish with lemon wedges, chopped fresh parsley (optional), and crusty bread for dipping (optional).

Tips:

- You can add other vegetables to the soup, such as chopped zucchini, chopped mushrooms, or chopped green beans.

- For a creamier soup, puree about half of the soup in a blender and return it to the pot.

- Leftover lentil soup can be stored in an airtight container in the refrigerator for up to 3 days. Reheat gently on the stovetop until warmed through.

Enjoy this hearty and satisfying lentil soup!

Vegetable Curry

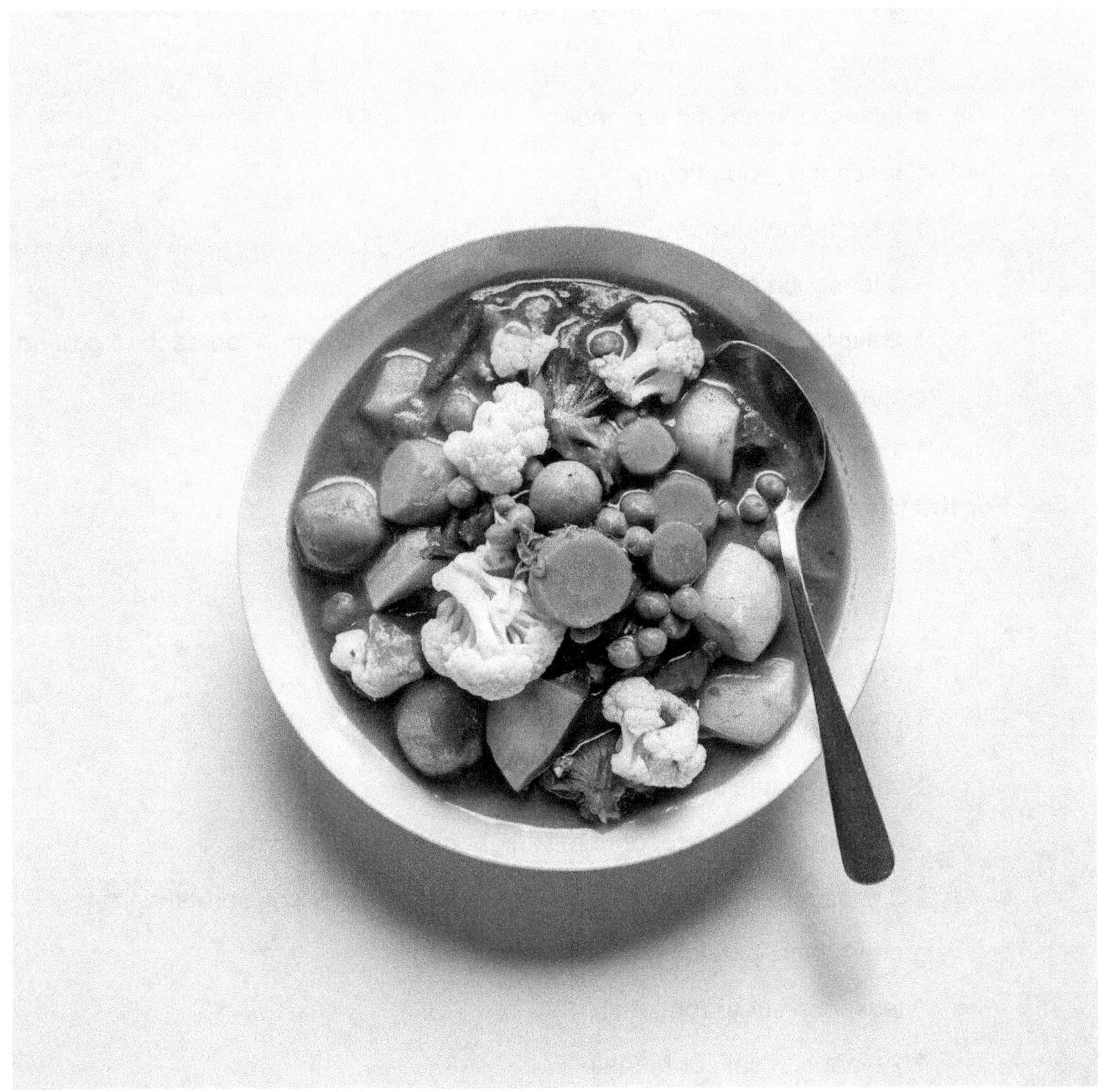

Ingredients:

- **For the Curry Paste (makes enough for 2-3 curries):**
    - 2 tablespoons vegetable oil
    - 1 large onion, chopped

- 2 cloves garlic, minced
- 1 inch ginger, peeled and minced
- 1 green chili pepper (optional, adjust for spice preference), seeded and chopped
- 1 tablespoon ground coriander
- 1 teaspoon ground cumin
- 1/2 teaspoon turmeric
- 1/4 teaspoon chili powder (optional)
- 1 teaspoon garam masala (or substitute with 1/2 teaspoon each of ground cinnamon, cloves, and cardamom)
- 1/2 teaspoon salt

- **For the Curry:**
  - 1 tablespoon vegetable oil
  - 1 medium onion, chopped
  - 1 bell pepper (any color), chopped
  - 1 (14.5-ounce) can diced tomatoes, undrained
  - 1 cup vegetable broth
  - 1 (13.5-ounce) can coconut milk (light or full-fat)
  - 2-3 cups mixed vegetables, chopped (such as broccoli florets, carrots, green beans, potatoes, cauliflower florets)
  - 1 teaspoon sugar (optional)
  - 1/2 teaspoon salt, or to taste
  - Freshly ground black pepper to taste
  - Cilantro leaves (chopped), for garnish (optional)
  - Cooked rice or naan bread, for serving

Instructions:

Preparation Time: 15 minutes **Cooking Time:** 30-35 minutes

1. **Make the Curry Paste (10 minutes):**
   - Heat vegetable oil in a skillet or pan over medium heat. Add the chopped onion and cook for 3-4 minutes, or until softened.
   - Add the minced garlic, ginger, and green chili pepper (if using). Cook for another minute, until fragrant.
   - Add the ground coriander, cumin, turmeric, chili powder (if using), garam masala, and salt. Stir and cook for 30 seconds, to toast the spices.
   - Transfer the mixture to a food processor or blender and grind into a smooth paste. You can add a little water if needed to help the blending process. Set aside.

2. **Sauté the Vegetables (5 minutes):**
   - Heat another tablespoon of vegetable oil in a large pot or Dutch oven over medium heat.
   - Add the chopped onion and bell pepper. Sauté for 5 minutes, or until softened.

3. **Add Curry Paste, Tomatoes, and Broth (5 minutes):**
   - Stir in the prepared curry paste, diced tomatoes (with their juices), and vegetable broth.
   - Bring to a simmer and cook for 5 minutes, allowing the flavors to meld.

4. **Add Coconut Milk and Vegetables (15-20 minutes):**
   - Stir in the coconut milk and your chosen mixed vegetables.
   - Simmer for 15-20 minutes, or until the vegetables are tender-crisp.

5. **Season and Serve (5 minutes):**
   - Season the curry with sugar (optional), salt, and freshly ground black pepper to taste.

- Garnish with chopped cilantro leaves (optional) and serve hot over cooked rice or with naan bread for dipping.

Tips:

- You can customize the vegetables in the curry based on your preferences. Other options include chopped zucchini, chopped eggplant, or chickpeas for added protein.
- Adjust the amount of chili pepper or chili powder to your desired level of spice.
- Leftover vegetable curry can be stored in an airtight container in the refrigerator for up to 3 days. Reheat gently on the stovetop until warmed through.

Enjoy this delicious and healthy vegetable curry!

Fish and Seafoods

Baked Salmon with Lemon Herb Crust

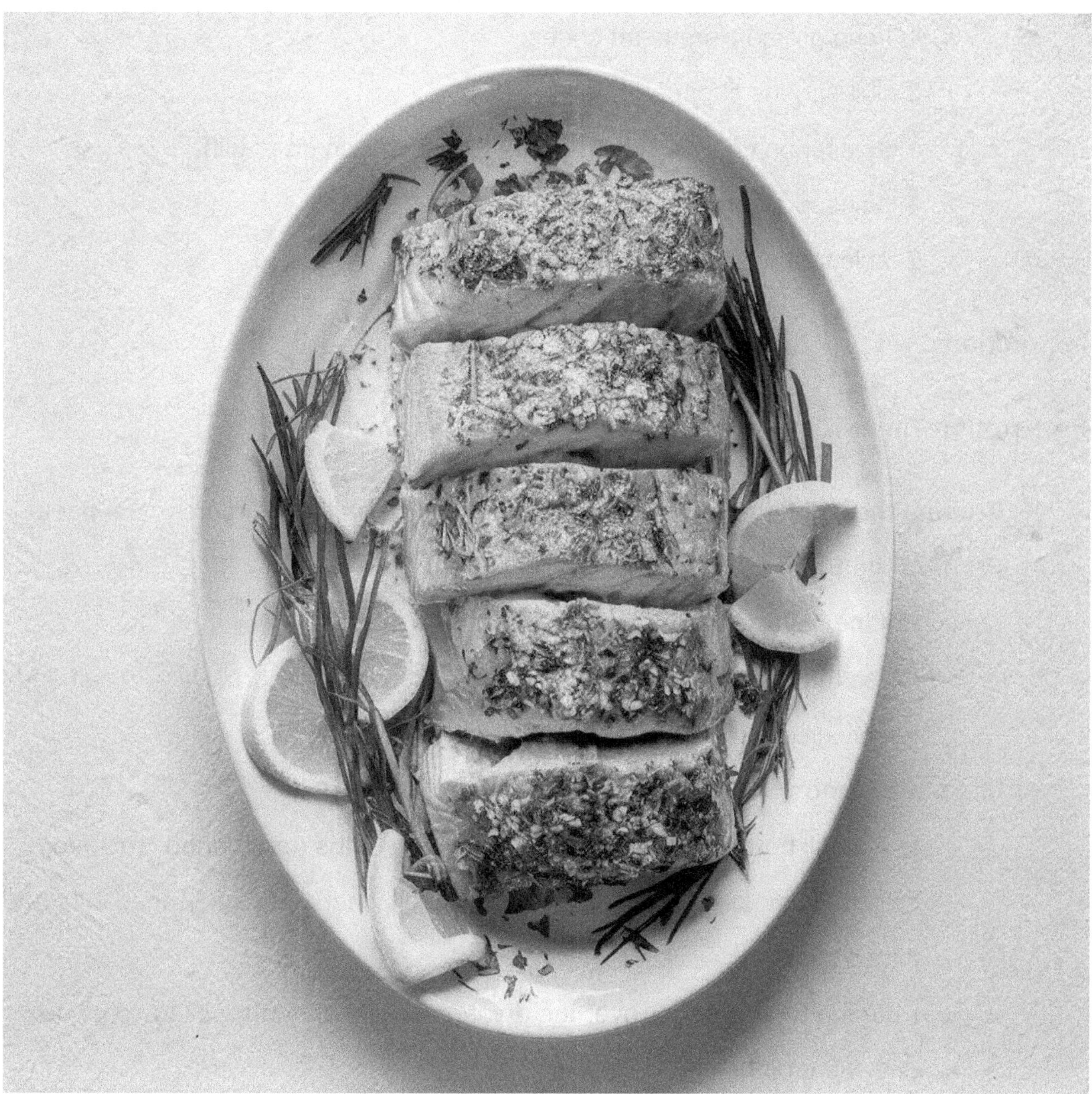

Ingredients:

- **For the Salmon:**

    - 2 salmon filets (each about 6 ounces)

    - 1 tablespoon olive oil

- ○ Salt and freshly ground black pepper to taste
- **For the Lemon Herb Crust:**
  - ○ 1/2 cup panko bread crumbs (or crushed crackers)
  - ○ 1/4 cup grated Parmesan cheese
  - ○ 2 tablespoons chopped fresh parsley
  - ○ 1 tablespoon chopped fresh dill (or 1/2 teaspoon dried dill)
  - ○ 1 tablespoon lemon zest
  - ○ 2 tablespoons melted butter

Instructions:

Preparation Time: 10 minutes **Cooking Time:** 12-15 minutes

1. **Preheat the oven to 400°F (200°C).** Line a baking sheet with parchment paper.
2. **Prepare the Salmon (5 minutes):**
   - ○ Pat the salmon fillets dry with paper towels.
   - ○ Brush the salmon fillets with olive oil and season generously with salt and freshly ground black pepper.
3. **Make the Lemon Herb Crust (5 minutes):**
   - ○ In a small bowl, combine the panko breadcrumbs (or crushed crackers), grated Parmesan cheese, chopped parsley, chopped dill (or dried dill), and lemon zest.
   - ○ Pour the melted butter over the dry ingredients and mix well to combine, until the crumbs are moistened.
4. **Assemble and Bake (12-15 minutes):**
   - ○ Spread the lemon herb crust evenly over the top of the seasoned salmon fillets.
   - ○ Place the salmon fillets on the prepared baking sheet.

- Bake for 12-15 minutes, or until the salmon is cooked through and the crust is golden brown. The internal temperature of the salmon should reach 145°F (63°C) for safe consumption.

5. **Serve (enjoy hot):**
   - Once cooked, remove the salmon from the oven and let it rest for a few minutes before serving.
   - Serve the baked salmon with lemon herb crust hot with your favorite sides, such as roasted vegetables, rice, or quinoa.

Tips:

- You can use fresh herbs like basil, thyme, or chives instead of parsley and dill in the crust.
- For a touch of spice, add a pinch of red pepper flakes to the crumb mixture.
- Salmon fillets can vary in thickness, so adjust the cooking time accordingly. Check for doneness by gently flaking the fish with a fork.
- Leftover baked salmon can be stored in an airtight container in the refrigerator for up to 3 days. Reheat gently in the oven or microwave until warmed through.

Enjoy this delicious and healthy baked salmon with lemon herb crust!

Shrimp Scampi with Zucchini Noodles

Here's a recipe for a light and flavorful Shrimp Scampi with Zucchini Noodles:

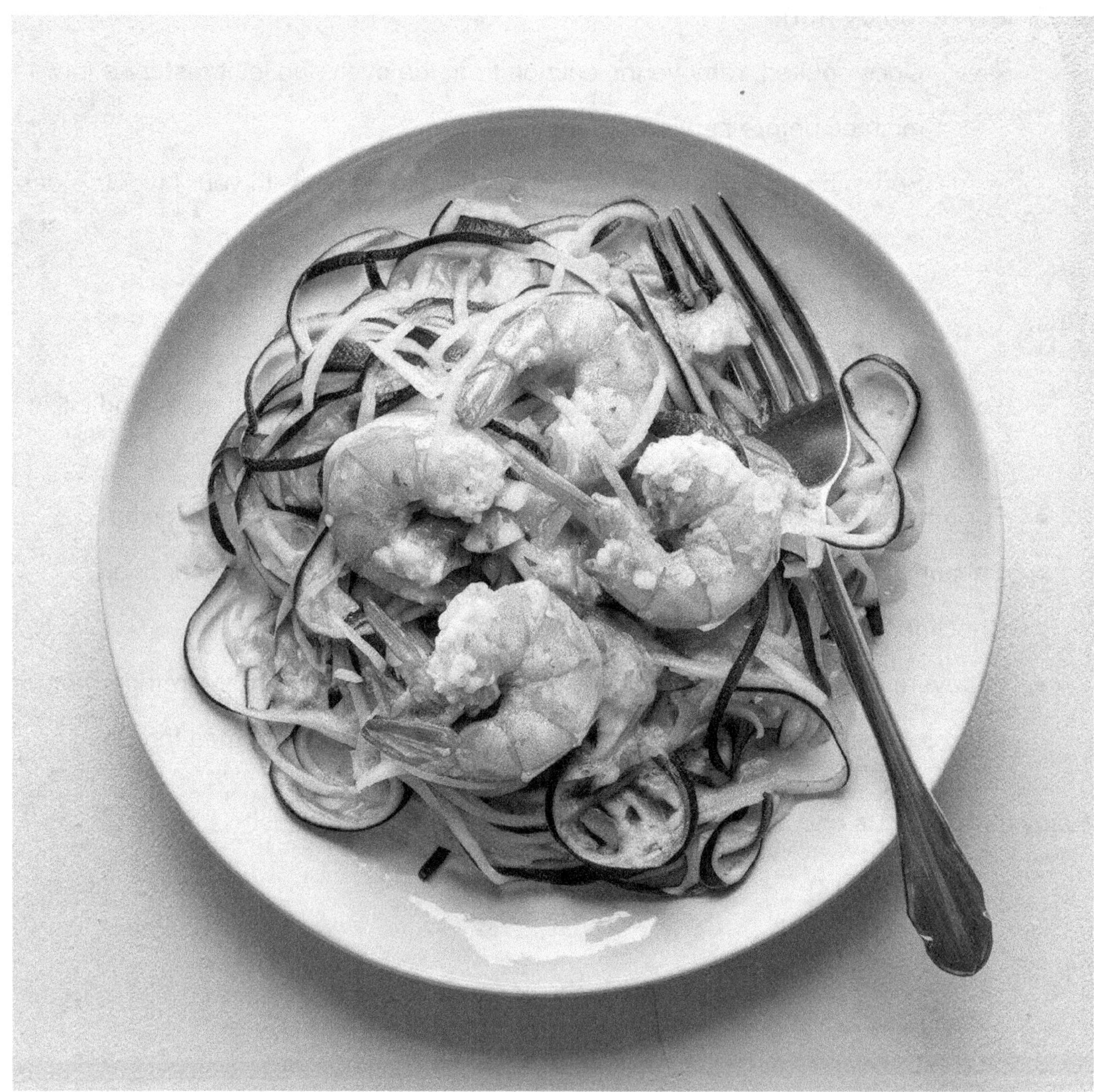

Ingredients:

- **For the Shrimp:**
  - 1 pound large shrimp, peeled and deveined
  - 1 tablespoon olive oil
  - 1/2 teaspoon dried oregano
  - 1/4 teaspoon garlic powder
  - Salt and freshly ground black pepper to taste
- **For the Zucchini Noodles:**
  - 2 medium zucchini (about 1 pound)
  - 1 tablespoon olive oil
  - 1/4 teaspoon salt
- **For the Garlic-Lemon Sauce:**
  - 2 tablespoons unsalted butter
  - 2 cloves garlic, minced
  - 1/4 cup dry white wine (or chicken broth)
  - 1/4 cup chopped fresh parsley
  - 1 tablespoon lemon juice
  - 1/4 teaspoon red pepper flakes (optional, adjust for spice preference)
  - Pinch of salt and freshly ground black pepper

Instructions:

Preparation Time: 15 minutes **Cooking Time:** 10-12 minutes

1. **Marinate the Shrimp (5 minutes, optional):**
   - In a medium bowl, combine the shrimp with olive oil, oregano, garlic powder, salt, and pepper. Toss to coat and marinate for at least 5 minutes

(while preparing the other ingredients) for added flavor, but this step is optional.

2. **Make the Zucchini Noodles (5 minutes):**
   - Using a spiralizer or julienne peeler, create zucchini noodles from the zucchini.
   - Heat olive oil in a large skillet or pan over medium heat. Add the zucchini noodles and cook for 2-3 minutes, stirring occasionally, until slightly softened but still crisp-tender. Season with salt and transfer the zucchini noodles to a bowl.

3. **Cook the Shrimp (3-4 minutes):**
   - In the same skillet used for the zucchini noodles, melt the butter over medium heat.
   - Add the shrimp (discarding the marinade if used) and cook for 2-3 minutes per side, or until pink and opaque. Be careful not to overcook the shrimp, as they will become rubbery.

4. **Make the Garlic-Lemon Sauce (2-3 minutes):**
   - Add the minced garlic to the pan with the cooked shrimp and cook for 30 seconds, until fragrant.
   - Pour in the white wine (or chicken broth) and bring to a simmer, scraping up any browned bits from the bottom of the pan.
   - Stir in the chopped parsley, lemon juice, red pepper flakes (if using), and a pinch of salt and pepper.
   - Let the sauce simmer for another minute to allow the flavors to meld.

5. **Serve (enjoy hot):**
   - Return the zucchini noodles to the pan with the shrimp and garlic-lemon sauce. Toss to coat the noodles evenly.

○ Serve immediately while hot. You can garnish with additional chopped fresh parsley or a squeeze of lemon juice (optional).

Tips:

- If you don't have a spiralizer, you can use a julienne peeler to create thin zucchini strips.
- You can adjust the amount of red pepper flakes to your desired level of spice.
- For a richer sauce, you can add a splash of heavy cream at the end.
- Leftover shrimp scampi with zucchini noodles can be stored in an airtight container in the refrigerator for up to 1 day. Reheat gently on the stovetop until warmed through, as the zucchini noodles may lose their crisp texture upon reheating.

Enjoy this delicious and healthy shrimp scampi with zucchini noodles!

Mediterranean Fish Stew

Here's a recipe for a flavorful and healthy Mediterranean Fish Stew:

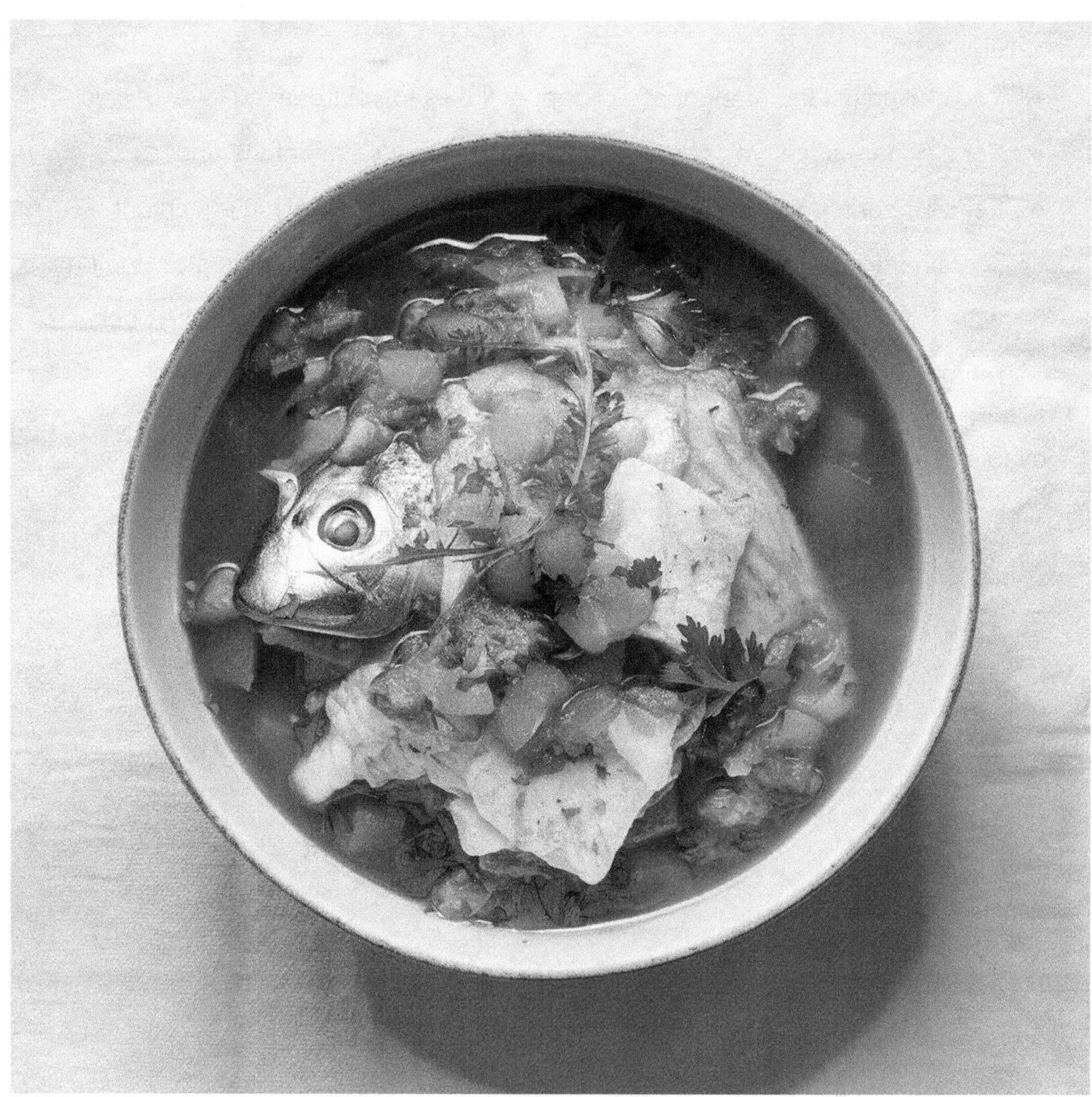

Ingredients:

- **For the Stew:**
    - 2 tablespoons olive oil
    - 1 onion, chopped
    - 2 celery stalks, chopped
    - 1 carrot, chopped
    - 2 cloves garlic, minced
    - 1 (14.5-ounce) can diced tomatoes, undrained
    - 1 cup dry white wine (or chicken broth)
    - 4 cups low-sodium vegetable broth
    - 1 teaspoon dried oregano
    - 1/2 teaspoon dried thyme
    - Pinch of red pepper flakes (optional)
    - 1 bay leaf
    - 1 pound skinless, white fish fillets (such as cod, halibut, or sea bass), cut into bite-sized pieces
    - 1/2 pound mussels, debearded (optional)
    - 1/2 pound shrimp, peeled and deveined (optional)
    - 1 cup chopped clams (optional)
    - 1/2 cup chopped fresh parsley
    - Salt and freshly ground black pepper to taste
- **For Serving (Optional):**
    - Crusty bread
    - Lemon wedges

Instructions:

Preparation Time: 15 minutes **Cooking Time:** 30-35 minutes

1. **Sauté the Vegetables (5 minutes):**
   - Heat olive oil in a large pot or Dutch oven over medium heat.
   - Add the chopped onion, celery, and carrot. Sauté for 5 minutes, or until softened.

2. **Add Garlic, Tomatoes, and Broth (5 minutes):**
   - Stir in the minced garlic and cook for another minute, until fragrant.
   - Add the diced tomatoes (with their juices), dry white wine (or chicken broth), vegetable broth, oregano, thyme, red pepper flakes (if using), and bay leaf.
   - Bring to a simmer and cook for 5 minutes, allowing the flavors to meld.

3. **Add Fish and Seafood (10-15 minutes):**
   - Gently add the fish pieces. If using mussels, clams, or shrimp, add them at this time as well.
   - Simmer for 10-15 minutes, or until the fish is cooked through and flaky, and the mussels and clams have opened (discard any unopened mussels or clams).

4. **Season and Serve (5 minutes):**
   - Stir in the chopped fresh parsley and season the stew with salt and freshly ground black pepper to taste.
   - Remove the bay leaf before serving.

5. **Serve (enjoy hot):**
   - Ladle the Mediterranean fish stew into bowls and serve hot with crusty bread for dipping and lemon wedges for squeezing over the stew (optional).

Tips:

- You can customize the fish and seafood in the stew based on your preferences and what's available. Other options include scallops, calamari, or even a combination of your favorites.
- If you don't have white wine, you can substitute it with an additional cup of vegetable broth.
- Leftover Mediterranean fish stew can be stored in an airtight container in the refrigerator for up to 2 days. Reheat gently on the stovetop until warmed through.

Enjoy this delicious and healthy taste of the Mediterranean!

Poultry and Meats

Honey Garlic Glazed Chicken

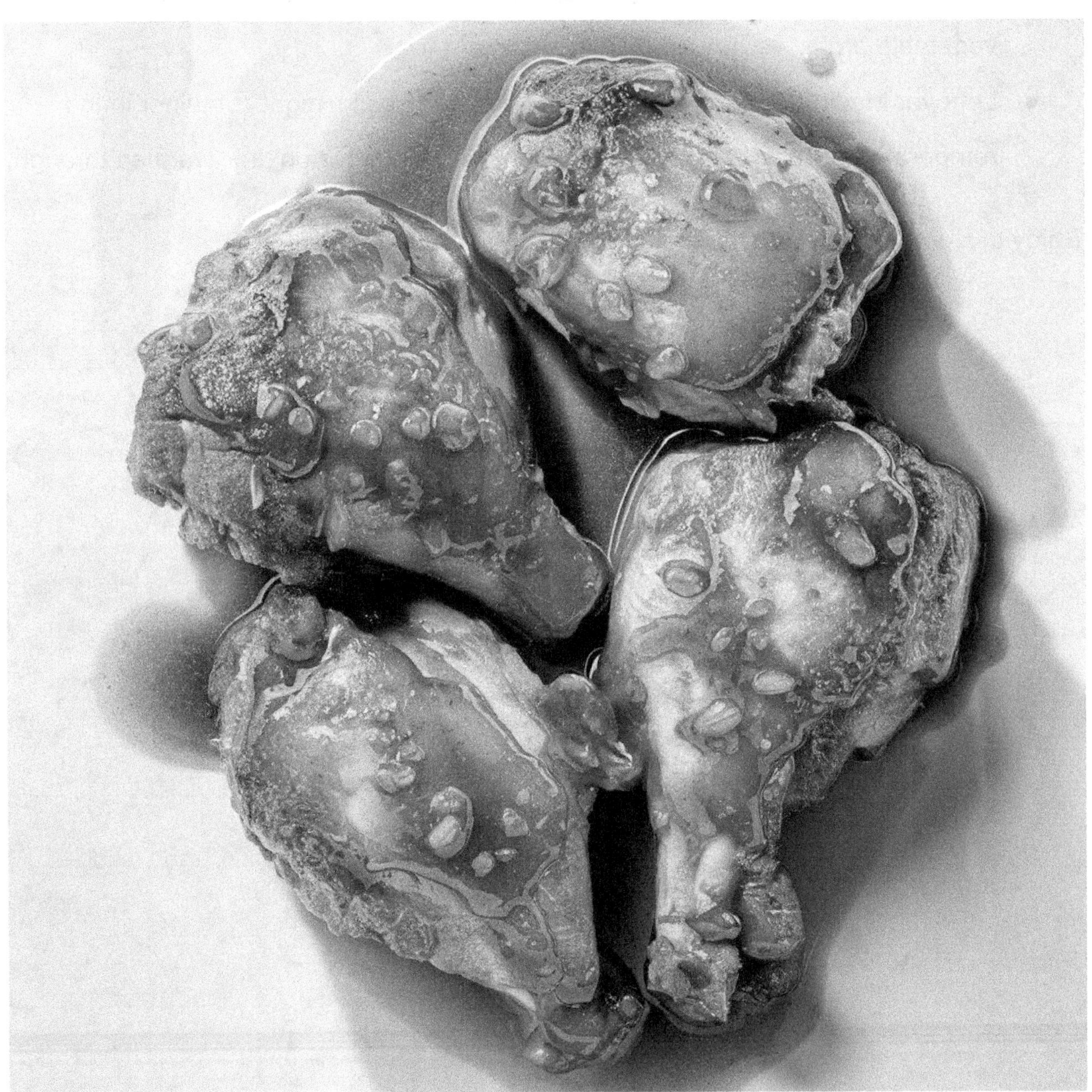

Ingredients:

- **For the Chicken:**
    - 2 boneless, skinless chicken breasts or thighs (about 1 pound total)

- 1/2 teaspoon salt

  - 1/4 teaspoon black pepper

  - 1 tablespoon olive oil

- **For the Honey Garlic Glaze:**

  - 1/3 cup honey

  - 2 tablespoons soy sauce

  - 1 tablespoon cornstarch (or arrowroot powder)

  - 1 tablespoon rice vinegar (or white vinegar)

  - 1 clove garlic, minced

  - 1/2 teaspoon ground ginger

Instructions:

Preparation Time: 10 minutes **Cooking Time:** 20-25 minutes

1. **Prep the Chicken (5 minutes):**

   - Pat the chicken breasts or thighs dry with paper towels.

   - Season them with salt and black pepper on both sides.

2. **Cook the Chicken (15-20 minutes):**

   - Heat olive oil in a large skillet or pan over medium heat.

   - Add the seasoned chicken and cook for 5-7 minutes per side, or until golden brown and cooked through. The internal temperature of the thickest part of the chicken should reach 165°F (74°C) for safe consumption.

3. **Make the Glaze (5 minutes):**

   - While the chicken cooks, whisk together the honey, soy sauce, cornstarch (or arrowroot powder), rice vinegar (or white vinegar), minced garlic, and ground ginger in a small bowl.

4. **Glaze the Chicken (5 minutes):**

   - Once the chicken is cooked through, transfer it to a plate.

   - Reduce the heat to medium-low and pour the prepared glaze into the pan where you cooked the chicken.

   - Bring the glaze to a simmer and cook for 2-3 minutes, or until the sauce thickens slightly.

5. **Serve (enjoy hot):**

   - Return the cooked chicken to the pan and coat it evenly with the thickened glaze.

   - Serve the honey garlic glazed chicken hot with your favorite sides, such as rice, noodles, or vegetables.

Tips:

- You can use chicken breasts or thighs for this recipe. Chicken thighs will result in a slightly more flavorful and tender chicken due to the higher fat content.

- If the glaze thickens too quickly, add a tablespoon or two of water to thin it out slightly.

- You can also thicken the glaze by simmering it for a longer time or by adding a cornstarch slurry (mix a teaspoon of cornstarch with a little water until smooth and stir it into the simmering glaze).

- Leftover honey garlic glazed chicken can be stored in an airtight container in the refrigerator for up to 3 days. Reheat gently in a pan with a little bit of sauce or water to prevent drying out.

Enjoy this delicious and easy Honey Garlic Glazed Chicken!

One-Pan Lemon Herb Roasted Chicken with Vegetables

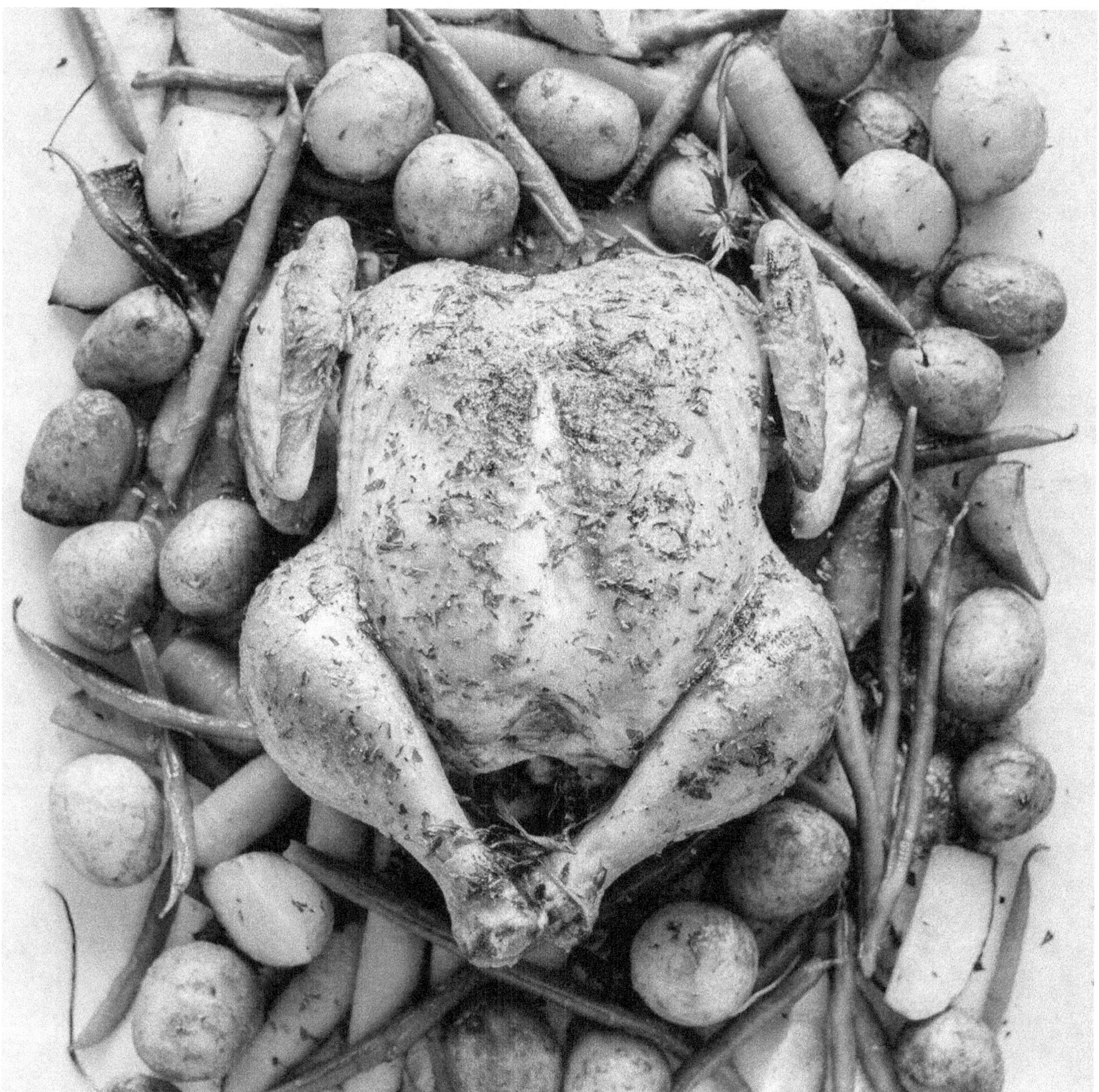

Ingredients:

- **For the Chicken:**

    - 1 whole chicken (around 3-4 pounds)

    - 1 tablespoon olive oil

- 1 lemon, halved
  - 2-3 sprigs fresh rosemary
  - 2-3 sprigs fresh thyme
  - Salt and freshly ground black pepper to taste
- **For the Vegetables:**
  - 1 pound potatoes (such as Yukon Gold or baby potatoes), cut into wedges
  - 1 pound carrots, peeled and cut into thick sticks
  - 1/2 onion, cut into wedges (optional)
  - 2 cloves garlic, minced (optional)

Instructions:

Preparation Time: 15 minutes **Cooking Time:** 1 hour - 1 hour 15 minutes

1. **Preheat the oven to 425°F (220°C).**
2. **Prep the Chicken (10 minutes):**
   - Pat the whole chicken dry with paper towels.
   - Drizzle the chicken cavity and skin with olive oil. Season generously with salt and pepper inside and out.
3. **Prep the Vegetables (5 minutes):**
   - In a large bowl, toss the potatoes, carrots, and onion wedges (if using) with olive oil, salt, and pepper.
4. **Assemble and Roast (55-75 minutes):**
   - Place the seasoned chicken in the center of a large rimmed baking sheet.
   - Stuff the lemon cavity with the rosemary and thyme sprigs.
   - Scatter the prepared vegetables around the chicken in the baking sheet.
   - Tuck the minced garlic cloves (if using) amongst the vegetables (optional).

- Roast for 55-75 minutes, or until the chicken is cooked through and the vegetables are tender-crisp. The internal temperature of the chicken thigh should reach 165°F (74°C) for safe consumption.

5. **Rest and Serve (enjoy hot):**
   - Once cooked, remove the pan from the oven and tent the chicken loosely with foil. Let it rest for 10-15 minutes before carving.
   - Carve the chicken and serve it with the roasted vegetables. You can drizzle any pan juices over the chicken and vegetables for extra flavor.

Tips:

- You can adjust the vegetables based on your preference. Other options include broccoli florets, Brussels sprouts, or bell peppers.
- If the vegetables start to brown too quickly, cover the pan loosely with foil during the last 15-20 minutes of roasting.
- Leftover roasted chicken and vegetables can be stored in an airtight container in the refrigerator for up to 3 days. Reheat gently in the oven or microwave until warmed through.

Enjoy this simple and delicious one-pan roasted chicken with vegetables!

Slow Cooker Beef Chili

Here's a delicious recipe for Slow Cooker Beef Chili, perfect for a hearty and comforting meal:

Ingredients:

- **For the Chili:**

    - 1 tablespoon olive oil
    - 1 onion, chopped
    - 1 green bell pepper, chopped (optional)
    - 2 cloves garlic, minced
    - 1 pound ground beef (80/20 lean-to-fat ratio is recommended for flavor)
    - 1 (28-ounce) can crushed tomatoes (undrained)
    - 1 (15-ounce) can kidney beans, drained and rinsed
    - 1 (15-ounce) can black beans, drained and rinsed
    - 1 (15-ounce) can pinto beans, drained and rinsed (optional)
    - 1 (14.5-ounce) can diced tomatoes with green chiles (undrained, optional)
    - 4 cups beef broth
    - 2 tablespoons chili powder
    - 1 tablespoon ground cumin
    - 1 teaspoon dried oregano
    - 1/2 teaspoon salt
    - 1/4 teaspoon black pepper
    - 1/4 teaspoon cayenne pepper (optional, adjust for spice preference)

- **For Serving (Optional):**

- o Shredded cheddar cheese
- o Chopped red onion
- o Sour cream
- o Chopped fresh cilantro
- o Lime wedges
- o Cornbread or crackers

Instructions:

Preparation Time: 15 minutes **Cooking Time:** 6-8 hours on low or 4-6 hours on high

1. **Sauté the Vegetables (optional, but adds flavor):**

   - o In a large skillet over medium heat, heat olive oil.
   - o Sauté the chopped onion and green bell pepper (if using) for 5 minutes, or until softened.
   - o Add the minced garlic and cook for another minute, until fragrant.
   - o Drain any excess grease from the pan.

2. **Transfer to Slow Cooker (or skip sauteing if preferred):**

   - o Transfer the sautéed vegetables (or the ground beef directly if you skipped sauteing) to your slow cooker.
   - o Add the ground beef, crushed tomatoes (undrained), drained and rinsed beans (kidney, black, and pinto beans if using), diced tomatoes with green chiles (undrained, optional), beef broth, chili powder, cumin, oregano, salt, black pepper, and cayenne pepper (optional).

3. **Slow Cook (6-8 hours on low or 4-6 hours on high):**

- Stir the ingredients in the slow cooker to combine.
- Cover and cook on low for 6-8 hours, or on high for 4-6 hours, or until the chili is thickened and the flavors have melded.

4. **Serve (enjoy hot):**

- Once cooked, ladle the chili into bowls and serve hot.
- You can garnish your chili with shredded cheddar cheese, chopped red onion, sour cream, chopped fresh cilantro, lime wedges (for squeezing), cornbread, or crackers (optional).

Tips:

- You can brown the ground beef in the same skillet you used to sauté the vegetables before adding it to the slow cooker for extra flavor.
- If you prefer a thicker chili, remove the lid during the last hour of cooking to allow some moisture to evaporate.
- You can adjust the spice level to your preference by adding more or less cayenne pepper.
- Leftover beef chili can be stored in an airtight container in the refrigerator for up to 5 days or frozen for up to 3 months. Reheat gently on the stovetop until warmed through.

Enjoy this delicious and easy slow cooker beef chili!

-

Broths and Smoothies

Vegetable Broth

Classic Vegetable Broth Recipe:

This recipe is a great base for many dishes and is simple to customize with your favorite vegetables and herbs.

Ingredients:

- 1 tablespoon olive oil (optional)
- 1 onion, chopped
- 2 carrots, chopped
- 2 celery stalks, chopped
- 2 cloves garlic, minced
- 1 teaspoon dried thyme
- 1 teaspoon dried parsley
- 1 bay leaf
- 8 cups water
- Salt and freshly ground black pepper to taste

Instructions:

Preparation Time: 10 minutes **Cooking Time:** 1 hour

1. **Optional Sauté (adds flavor):**
   - In a large pot or Dutch oven, heat olive oil over medium heat (optional).
   - Add the chopped onion, carrots, and celery. Sauté for 5 minutes, or until softened.
2. **Add Remaining Ingredients:**

    o Add the minced garlic, dried thyme, dried parsley, and bay leaf to the pot.

    o Pour in the water and bring to a boil.

3. **Simmer and Season:**

    o Reduce heat to low and simmer for 1 hour, or until the vegetables are tender and the flavors have melded.

    o Season the broth with salt and freshly ground black pepper to taste.

4. **Strain and Serve:**

    o Strain the broth through a fine-mesh sieve to remove the vegetables and herbs.

    o Serve the vegetable broth hot or store it in an airtight container in the refrigerator for up to 5 days or freeze for up to 3 months.

Tips:

- You can customize this recipe by adding other vegetables such as mushrooms, potatoes, or tomatoes.
- Feel free to experiment with different herbs and spices, such as rosemary, oregano, or bay leaves.
- If you prefer a richer flavor, you can roast the vegetables in the oven before adding them to the pot.
- Leftover vegetable broth can be used in soups, stews, sauces, gravies, or rice dishes.

Vegetable Broth from Scraps:

This recipe is a great way to reduce food waste and create a flavorful broth.

Ingredients:

- Vegetable scraps, such as onion peels, carrot ends, celery trimmings, mushroom stems, herb sprigs, tomato cores, etc.
- 8 cups water
- Optional: 1 tablespoon olive oil
- Salt and freshly ground black pepper to taste

Instructions:

Preparation Time: 5 minutes **Cooking Time:** 1 hour

1. **Gather Scraps:**
   - Collect vegetable scraps from your cooking throughout the week.
2. **Simmer the Scraps:**
   - In a large pot or Dutch oven, heat olive oil over medium heat (optional).
   - Add the collected vegetable scraps.
   - Pour in the water and bring to a boil.
3. **Simmer and Season:**
   - Reduce heat to low and simmer for 1 hour, or until the flavors have melded.
   - Season the broth with salt and freshly ground black pepper to taste.
4. **Strain and Store:**
   - Strain the broth through a fine-mesh sieve to remove the vegetable scraps.
   - Serve the vegetable broth hot or store it in an airtight container in the refrigerator for up to 5 days or freeze for up to 3 months.

Tips:

- Avoid scraps that have begun to mold or rot.

- You can add a bay leaf or other herbs for additional flavor.

- This broth may not be as strong flavored as a broth made with fresh vegetables, so you may need to use more in your recipes.

Enjoy these delicious and versatile vegetable broth recipes!

Chicken Broth

Here's a recipe for a classic and flavorful Chicken Broth:

Ingredients:

- **For the Broth:**
    - 1 whole chicken (around 3-4 pounds), skin-on (optional)
    - 1 onion, quartered
    - 2 carrots, peeled and roughly chopped
    - 2 celery stalks, roughly chopped
    - 2-3 cloves garlic, peeled
    - 1 teaspoon dried thyme
    - 1 teaspoon dried parsley
    - 1 bay leaf
    - 10 whole black peppercorns
    - 12 cups water
    - Salt to taste

- **Optional Vegetables (for additional flavor):**

- ○ 1 parsnip, peeled and roughly chopped

- ○ 1 leek, white and light green parts only, halved and rinsed

Instructions:

Preparation Time: 15 minutes **Cooking Time:** 2-3 hours

1. **Prep the Chicken and Vegetables (10 minutes):**
   - ○ Rinse the chicken under cold water and pat it dry with paper towels. You can leave the skin on or remove it for a less fatty broth.
   - ○ Roughly chop the onion, carrots, and celery. Peel the garlic cloves.

2. **Combine Ingredients and Bring to a Boil (5 minutes):**
   - ○ In a large pot or Dutch oven, combine the chicken, vegetables (including optional vegetables), herbs (thyme, parsley, bay leaf), peppercorns, and water.
   - ○ Bring the mixture to a boil over medium-high heat.

3. **Simmer and Skim (1 hour):**
   - ○ Once boiling, reduce heat to low and simmer gently for 1-2 hours, skimming any foam or fat that rises to the surface with a spoon.

4. **Season and Strain (1-2 hours):**
   - ○ After simmering for 1-2 hours, or until the chicken is cooked through (the internal temperature of the thickest part of the thigh should reach 165°F (74°C) for safe consumption), remove the pot from heat.
   - ○ Season the broth with salt to taste.
   - ○ Carefully remove the chicken and vegetables from the broth using a slotted spoon. You can shred the chicken meat for later use in soups or stews (optional).
   - ○ Strain the broth through a fine-mesh sieve into a clean pot or container.

5. **Cool, Store, or Use (enjoy hot):**
   - Let the broth cool slightly before storing or using. You can skim off any additional fat that rises to the surface after cooling.
   - Store the broth in an airtight container in the refrigerator for up to 5 days or freeze for up to 3 months.
   - Use the chicken broth as a base for soups, stews, sauces, gravies, or rice dishes. You can also enjoy it hot as a comforting beverage.

Tips:

- Roasting the chicken and vegetables before adding them to the pot can add a deeper flavor to the broth.
- You can adjust the amount of water depending on how concentrated you want your broth to be. Reduce the water by a couple of cups for a stronger broth, or add more water for a milder flavor.
- If you prefer a clearer broth, you can clarify it by whisking in a few egg whites before bringing it back to a simmer. Once the egg whites coagulate and rise to the surface, strain the broth again.
- Leftover cooked chicken from the broth can be used in various dishes, such as soups, stews, salads, or sandwiches.

Enjoy this delicious and homemade chicken broth recipe!

Green Smoothie

Ingredients:

- **For the Base:**
    - 1 cup unsweetened almond milk (or other plant-based milk of your choice)
    - 1/2 banana, frozen (adds sweetness and creaminess)
    - 1 handful (about 1 cup) spinach or kale (fresh or frozen)
- **For the Flavor:**
    - 1/2 cup frozen mango or pineapple (or other fruits of your choice)
    - 1 tablespoon chopped fresh ginger (optional, for a kick)
    - 1 teaspoon ground flaxseed (optional, for added fiber and nutrients)
    - 1/2 cup plain Greek yogurt (optional, for extra protein and creaminess)
    - Honey or maple syrup (optional, to taste)

Instructions:

Preparation Time: 5 minutes **Servings:** 1

1. **Blend the Base:**
    - Add the unsweetened almond milk, frozen banana piece, and spinach or kale to a blender.
2. **Add Flavor Boosters (optional):**
    - Add your chosen fruits (mango, pineapple, etc.), ginger (if using), flaxseed (if using), and Greek yogurt (if using).
3. **Blend Until Smooth:**

- ○ Blend all ingredients on high speed until you have a smooth and creamy consistency. You may need to use the tamper to push down the ingredients if your blender is struggling.

4. **Taste and Adjust (optional):**
   - ○ Taste your smoothie and adjust the sweetness to your preference by adding honey or maple syrup (optional).

5. **Enjoy!**
   - ○ Pour the green smoothie into a glass and enjoy it immediately for maximum freshness.

Tips:

- You can customize this recipe with different fruits, vegetables, and add-ins to create your own flavor combinations. Here are some ideas:
  - ○ **Fruits:** Berries (fresh or frozen), peaches, kiwi, pear, avocado (for a creamier texture).
  - ○ **Vegetables:** Celery, cucumber (for a more refreshing drink).
  - ○ **Add-ins:** Protein powder, nut butter, chia seeds, spirulina powder (for extra nutrients), fresh mint or basil leaves.
- If you don't have fresh spinach or kale, you can use frozen spinach or kale for convenience.
- Frozen fruit helps create a thicker and colder smoothie. You can use fresh fruit if preferred, but you may need to add ice cubes for a chilled drink.
- Start with less liquid and add more if needed to achieve your desired consistency.
- Leftover smoothie can be stored in an airtight container in the refrigerator for up to 1 day, but the flavor and texture may deteriorate.

Enjoy this healthy and delicious green smoothie!

Desserts

Dark Chocolate Avocado Mousse

- This decadent mousse is surprisingly healthy and made with nourishing ingredients like avocado and dark chocolate. It's a great source of healthy fats and antioxidants, and it can help regulate blood sugar levels.

Here's a recipe for this delicious mousse:

Ingredients:

- 2 ripe avocados, pitted and peeled
- ¾ cup unsweetened cocoa powder
- ¼ cup honey or maple syrup
- ¼ cup milk (dairy-free or regular milk)
- 1 teaspoon vanilla extract
- Pinch of salt

Instructions:

1. In a blender, combine the avocados, cocoa powder, honey or maple syrup, milk, vanilla extract, and salt. Blend until smooth and creamy.
2. Taste and adjust sweetness as desired.
3. Pour the mousse into individual serving cups or a small bowl.
4. Refrigerate for at least 30 minutes before serving.

Baked Apples with Berries and Nuts

- This is a classic and healthy dessert that's perfect for PCOS patients. Baked apples are a good source of fiber and antioxidants, and they can help regulate blood sugar levels. The berries and nuts add extra flavor, fiber, and healthy fats.

Here's a recipe for this delicious and nutritious dessert:

Ingredients:

- 4 apples (such as Gala, Fuji, or Honeycrisp)
- 1 cup mixed berries (fresh or frozen)
- ¼ cup chopped walnuts or pecans
- 2 tablespoons unsalted butter, melted
- 1 tablespoon ground cinnamon
- ¼ teaspoon ground nutmeg
- Pinch of salt

Instructions:

1. Preheat the oven to 375°F (190°C).
2. Wash the apples and core them, leaving the bottoms intact.
3. In a medium bowl, combine the berries, nuts, melted butter, cinnamon, nutmeg, and salt.
4. Stuff the apple cores with the berry mixture.
5. Place the apples in a baking dish and bake for 30-35 minutes, or until the apples are tender and cooked through.
6. Serve warm or at room temperature.

Chia Seed Pudding

- Chia seed pudding is a trendy and healthy dessert that's perfect for PCOS patients. Chia seeds are a good source of fiber, protein, and healthy fats, and they can help regulate blood sugar levels. This pudding is also very versatile and can be customized with different flavors and toppings.

Here's a recipe for this nutritious and satisfying dessert:

Ingredients:

- ½ cup chia seeds
- 1 cup unsweetened almond milk (or other plant-based milk)
- ¼ cup yogurt (dairy-free or regular yogurt)
- 2 tablespoons honey or maple syrup
- 1 teaspoon vanilla extract
- Pinch of salt
- Toppings (optional): Fresh berries, chopped nuts, shredded coconut, sliced banana

Instructions:

1. In a bowl or jar, whisk together the chia seeds, almond milk, yogurt, honey or maple syrup, vanilla extract, and salt.
2. Cover the bowl or jar and refrigerate for at least 2 hours, or overnight for a thicker pudding.
3. When ready to serve, stir the pudding and portion it into individual serving cups or bowls.
4. Top with your favorite toppings, such as fresh berries, chopped nuts, shredded coconut, or sliced banana.

Chapter 4: Lifestyle Tips

Exercise and Movement

1. Cardio with moderate intensity

Brisk walking,

jogging,

swimming,

cycling,

dancing.

- **Movement Tips:** Aim for at least 30 minutes of moderate-intensity cardio most days of the week. This will help improve insulin sensitivity and manage blood sugar levels. You can break it down into smaller chunks throughout the day if needed (e.g., 3 sessions of 10 minutes each).

2. Strength Training:

Bodyweight squats,

lunges,

push-ups (modifications can be done),

resistance band exercises,

weightlifting with lighter weights and higher repetitions.

- **Movement Tips:** Focus on building strength in all major muscle groups (legs, core, back, chest, shoulders) 2-3 times a week. Strength training helps manage weight, improve insulin sensitivity, and build bone density.

3. Yoga or Pilates:

> Downward-facing dog,
>
> warrior poses,
>
> bridge pose,
>
> planks,
>
> cat-cow stretches,
>
> pelvic tilts.

- **Movement Tips:** Yoga and Pilates combine elements of strength training, flexibility, and mindfulness. They can help improve insulin sensitivity, manage stress (a factor in PCOS), and promote relaxation.

4. High-Intensity Interval Training (HIIT) - Can be done in moderation:

> Burpees,
>
> jumping jacks,
>
> jumping squats,
>
> mountain climbers (with modifications if needed).
>
> Short bursts of intense activity followed by rest periods.

- **Movement Tips:** HIIT workouts can be a time-efficient way to improve insulin sensitivity and burn calories. However, for PCOS patients, it's crucial to listen to your body and start slowly, incorporating short HIIT sessions (10-15 minutes) 1-2 times a week initially.

5. Low-Impact Activities:

> Walking,
>
> stationary cycling,

water aerobics,

gentle yoga or Pilates modifications.

- **Movement Tips:** Low-impact activities are a great way to stay active, especially on days when your body needs more recovery or experiences joint pain. They can help improve circulation and overall fitness.

General Tips:

- **Warm-up before each workout:** This helps prepare your muscles and joints for exercise and reduces the risk of injury.
- **Cool down after each workout:** This helps your body return to its resting state and reduces muscle soreness.
- **Listen to your body:** Don't push yourself too hard, especially when starting a new exercise routine. Take rest days when needed.
- **Consult a healthcare professional:** It's important to get clearance from your doctor before starting any new exercise program, especially if you have any underlying health conditions. They can help create a personalized exercise plan that's safe and effective for you.

Remember, consistency is key! Aim for a combination of these exercises throughout the week to manage your PCOS symptoms and improve your overall health.

Stress Management Techniques

Here are 7 useful and detailed stress management techniques you can incorporate into your daily life:

1. **Mindfulness and Meditation:**

- **What it is:** Mindfulness involves focusing your awareness on the present moment without judgment. Meditation is a practice that cultivates mindfulness. There are many different meditation techniques, but some popular ones include focusing on your breath, repeating a mantra (a calming word or phrase), or body scan meditation (focusing attention on different parts of your body).
- **Benefits:** Mindfulness and meditation can help reduce stress hormones, improve focus, and promote relaxation.
- **How to do it:** There are many guided meditations available online and in apps. You can start with just a few minutes a day and gradually increase the duration as you become more comfortable.

2. **Relaxation Techniques:**

- **What it is:** Relaxation techniques encompass various practices that help reduce muscle tension and calm the mind and body. Some examples include progressive muscle relaxation (tensing and releasing different muscle groups), deep breathing exercises, and visualization (imagining yourself in a peaceful setting).
- **Benefits:** Relaxation techniques can lower blood pressure, slow your heart rate, and ease anxiety.
- **How to do it:** There are many resources available online and in apps to learn different relaxation techniques.

3. **Regular Exercise:**

- **What it is:** Physical activity is a powerful stress reliever. Exercise releases endorphins, hormones that have mood-boosting and pain-relieving effects.
- **Benefits:** Exercise can improve sleep quality, reduce stress hormones, and increase energy levels.

- **How to do it:** Aim for at least 30 minutes of moderate-intensity exercise most days of the week. You can break it down into shorter sessions throughout the day if needed. Find activities you enjoy, like brisk walking, dancing, swimming, or cycling.

4. **Healthy Sleep Habits:**

- **What it is:** Chronic sleep deprivation can significantly worsen stress levels. Aim for 7-8 hours of quality sleep each night.

- **Benefits:** Adequate sleep improves concentration, mood regulation, and overall physical and mental health.

- **How to do it:** Establish a regular sleep schedule, go to bed and wake up at consistent times even on weekends. Create a relaxing bedtime routine, such as taking a warm bath or reading a book. Make sure your bedroom is dark, quiet, and cool.

5. **Time Management and Organization:**

- **What it is:** Feeling overwhelmed by tasks can be a major stressor. Effective time management and organization can help you feel more in control.

- **Benefits:** Good time management skills allow you to prioritize tasks, meet deadlines, and reduce feelings of being overwhelmed.

- **How to do it:** Create to-do lists, set realistic goals, and schedule time for important tasks. Break down large projects into smaller, more manageable steps. Learn to delegate tasks when possible.

6. **Connecting with Others:**

- **What it is:** Social support is crucial for managing stress. Having strong social connections can provide a sense of belonging, reduce loneliness, and offer emotional support during challenging times.

- **Benefits:** Spending time with loved ones can help you feel less alone, boost your mood, and provide a sense of perspective.

- **How to do it:** Schedule regular time for friends and family. Join a club or group activity that interests you. Volunteer your time to a cause you care about.

7. **Healthy Lifestyle Choices:**

- **What it is:** Taking care of your physical health can significantly impact your stress levels. This includes eating a balanced diet, limiting alcohol and caffeine intake, and staying hydrated.

- **Benefits:** A healthy lifestyle can improve your energy levels, mood, and overall well-being, making you more resilient to stress.

- **How to do it:** Eat plenty of fruits, vegetables, and whole grains. Limit processed foods, sugary drinks, and unhealthy fats. Drink plenty of water throughout the day.

Remember, finding the right stress management techniques depends on your individual needs and preferences. Experiment with different approaches and find what works best for you. You can also combine several techniques for a more comprehensive approach to stress management.

Prioritizing Sleep and Rest

In our fast-paced world, sleep and rest often take a back seat. We push ourselves to work longer hours, juggle multiple commitments, and stay glued to our screens. But skimping on sleep has a significant impact on our physical and mental well-being. Prioritizing sleep and rest is not a luxury, but a necessity for optimal functioning.

Why Sleep and Rest Matter

Sleep is not simply a period of inactivity; it's a vital biological process essential for:

- **Physical Repair and Restoration:** During sleep, your body repairs tissues, strengthens the immune system, and releases hormones that regulate growth and development.
- **Cognitive Function:** Sleep is crucial for memory consolidation, learning, and decision-making. When sleep-deprived, you experience difficulty concentrating, increased forgetfulness, and impaired judgment.
- **Mood Regulation:** Sleep deprivation disrupts the production of neurotransmitters like serotonin and dopamine, which affect mood and emotional well-being. It can increase irritability, anxiety, and symptoms of depression.
- **Physical Health:** Chronic sleep deprivation is linked to various health problems, including obesity, heart disease, diabetes, and high blood pressure.

Rest goes beyond sleep and encompasses activities that allow your body and mind to de-stress and recharge. This may include taking breaks throughout the day, engaging in relaxation techniques, or simply doing activities you find enjoyable.

The Benefits of Prioritizing Sleep and Rest:

- **Enhanced Energy Levels:** Feeling tired throughout the day is a common consequence of sleep deprivation. Prioritizing sleep leads to increased energy and improved stamina for daily activities.
- **Improved Concentration and Focus:** Sleep-deprived individuals struggle to concentrate and have difficulty focusing on tasks. Getting enough sleep allows for better focus, clearer thinking, and enhanced problem-solving abilities.
- **Boosted Mood:** Adequate sleep promotes the production of mood-regulating neurotransmitters, leading to a more positive outlook, reduced stress, and better emotional resilience.
- **Stronger Immune System:** Sleep plays a vital role in immune function. When well-rested, your body is better equipped to fight off infections and illnesses.
- **Reduced Risk of Chronic Diseases:** Studies have shown a correlation between chronic sleep deprivation and an increased risk of developing chronic diseases like heart disease, diabetes, and obesity.
- **Improved Physical Performance:** Both sleep and rest are essential for athletes and anyone who engages in physical activity. Adequate rest allows for muscle recovery, improved coordination, and enhanced performance.

Tips for Prioritizing Sleep and Rest:

- **Establish a Regular Sleep Schedule: Go to bed and wake up at consistent times, even on weekends. This helps regulate your body's natural sleep-wake cycle.**

- **Create a Relaxing Bedtime Routine: Wind down before bed with calming activities like reading a book, taking a warm bath, or practicing relaxation techniques. Avoid screens for at least an hour before bedtime as the blue light emitted can interfere with sleep.**

- **Optimize Your Sleep Environment: Ensure your bedroom is dark, quiet, cool, and clutter-free. Invest in a comfortable mattress and pillows to promote better sleep quality.**

- **Develop a Relaxing Morning Routine: Avoid hitting the snooze button and start your day with calming activities like gentle stretches, meditation, or spending time in nature.**

- **Limit Caffeine and Alcohol: While caffeine can provide a temporary energy boost, it can disrupt sleep patterns later in the day. Similarly, excessive alcohol consumption can worsen sleep quality.**

- **Regular Exercise: Engage in regular physical activity, but avoid strenuous workouts close to bedtime. Exercise promotes better sleep but needs time for the body to wind down afterwards.**

- **Manage Stress: Chronic stress can significantly impact sleep quality. Practice relaxation techniques like deep breathing, meditation, or yoga to manage stress levels.**

- **Listen to Your Body: Pay attention to your body's natural sleep cues. If you feel tired after 7-8 hours of sleep, consult a doctor to rule out any underlying sleep disorders.**

- **Schedule Rest Throughout the Day:** Take short breaks throughout your workday to stretch, walk around, or simply close your eyes and relax.

- **Engage in Restful Activities:** Make time for activities you find enjoyable and relaxing, whether it's reading, spending time in nature, listening to calming music, or spending time with loved ones.

Remember, prioritizing sleep and rest is an investment in your overall health and well-being. By making small changes to your daily routine and incorporating strategies for relaxation, you can experience the numerous benefits of a good night's sleep and a well-rested mind and body.